THE COMPLETE KETOGENIC DIET FOR BEGINNERS

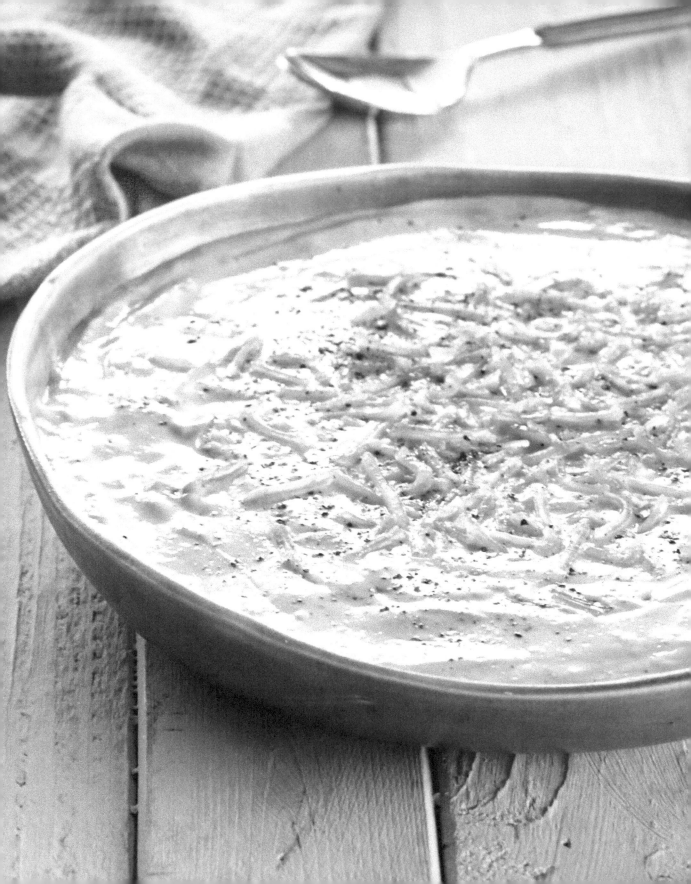

THE COMPLETE KETOGENIC DIET FOR BEGINNERS

Your Essential Guide to Living the Keto Lifestyle

AMY RAMOS

ROCKRIDGE PRESS

CONTENTS

FOREWORD

MY ITALIAN RELATIVES STILL SCOFF AT ME WHEN I SKIP THE BREAD AT DINNER. They say, "But it's the weekend! Nobody diets on the weekend!"

To be clear, the ketogenic diet doesn't break for weekends. It doesn't flip its hair and sneak candy from the bowl while the cauliflower isn't looking. Staying in ketosis is a full-time job, but after you break through your carb withdrawals in week one, you're going to be so pumped with energy that you'll be slaying doughnuts and mashed potatoes with the sword of shame.

Over the past decade, I've talked to people from all walks of life who are on the ketogenic diet. While the diet has been used to treat epilepsy informally since at least 500 BC, it's been recommended by the medical community since the 1920s.[1] But most commonly, people reach out to me for a host of other reasons, not just because they have epilepsy and need to change their diet. I've spoken with patients who are using the ketogenic diet as recommended by the nutritionist at their cancer centers, and I've even met people who have used the diet to combat anxiety and depression. In addition to weight loss, going keto helped me fight chronic vertigo, which prevented me from driving for three years.

Glucose imbalance, the result of eating a diet heavy in breads, sugars, starches, and pasta, is said to be harmful to the brain, so it's no wonder when glucose is replaced with ketones. A ketogenic diet can help to restore brain function for people who suffer with dementia and Alzheimer's disease (also sometimes referred to as type 3 diabetes[2]). A brain that isn't hopped up on sugar is a happy brain!

This book you're about to read is an excellent guide to following a ketogenic diet, no matter how much weight you want to lose, or how much of your life you want to regain.

---

1 https://www.ncbi.nlm.nih.gov/pubmed/19049574

2 https://www.ncbi.nlm.nih.gov/pmc/articles/PMC2769828/

Whenever you approach a diet, you should go into it thinking that you're adapting to a healthier lifestyle. However, in the ketogenic community, you'll often find forums and Facebook groups riddled with ketogenic junkfood (Take your McDonald's burger, throw away the bun, and flip it inside out! Yeah! Keto-friendly!). What I love about this book is that it brings healthy ingredients to the forefront, without being snobby. This diet is heavy on fat, so why not choose healthy ones that provide additional health benefits, like coconut oil, ghee, and avocado? Hang those highly processed oils, like vegetable oils and soybean oils, out to dry.

In addition, you'll find specific examples throughout this book; for example, berries are a-ok, but you shouldn't eat bananas because they contain more than your daily intake of carbohydrates. And chapter 2, on setting up your kitchen, includes a crucial set of equipment for making delicious ketogenic meals (a cast-iron pan, especially!).

The section on keto-friendly alternatives is particularly useful, because you may not know that a cup of milk has 13 net carbs, while unsweetened almond milk contains zero carbs (and is just as tasty!). I've known numerous people who assumed they can eat rice on this diet (it's like Paleo, right?) and I need to explain that rice has 44 net carbs per (cooked) cup. When you tell them you're shooting for less than 20 net carbs per day, it just about blows their mind.

And probably my favorite part of the book? Every recipe is 6 carbs! That's some no-brainer type of keto stuff I can get behind. Enjoy this book and your path to ketogenic wellness!

Amanda C. Hughes
Keto Cook at WickedStuffed.com
Author of *Keto Life* and *The Wicked Good Ketogenic Diet Cookbook*

INTRODUCTION

WITH THIS BOOK AS YOUR GUIDE, you can easily make the lifestyle change millions of other people have successfully made. You can feel and look great by eating food that's healthy, natural, and delicious. It will benefit your mental and physical health and provide constant energy throughout your day.

To be successful, you'll need to understand the very basics of your body and dieting.

Low-fat, low-calorie, gluten-free, Atkins, Weight Watchers, South Beach . . . the list of diets goes on. Most require you to starve yourself, eat bland, uninspiring food, strictly count calories, or go through various induction phases. The major problem with these diets is that they aren't always nutritionally sound and they're certainly not satisfying. That's simply not safe or sustainable. They are not a lifestyle.

What the more successful diets have in common is the reduction of foods rich in carbohydrates. Studies show that people who eat low-carb diets and don't reduce calories lose more weight than people who eat low-fat diets and also reduce calories. In addition, low-carb dieters generally show more improvement for important health indicators like triglyceride, blood sugar, and insulin levels, and more.

This all comes down to how your body works. When you eat carbs, your body breaks them down into glucose, a simple sugar, which quickly and significantly raises your blood sugar levels. Then you produce insulin to reduce this spike in blood sugar. After years and years of this cycle, your body will need to produce more insulin at once to achieve the same results. You can quickly become insulin resistant, and very commonly this resistance turns into prediabetes, metabolic syndrome, and, eventually, type 2 diabetes.

According to the American Diabetes Association's (ADA's) 2012 data, more than 1 in 3 adults in the United States have prediabetes and nearly 1 in 10 have type 2 diabetes. Data from the Centers for Disease Control and Prevention (CDC) shows the number of obese adults in the United States has spiked since the 1980s from 15 percent to 35 percent of all adults ages 20 to 74. This increase can only be attributed to a change in diet on a national scale.

The US Department of Agriculture (USDA) first released their Dietary Guidelines in 1980, and they recommended that fats and oils be heavily reduced along with sweets while carbohydrates should account for most of your daily food consumption. Soon after they released the Food Pyramid Guide, which placed carbs into the largest section of the pyramid and recommended that you eat 6 to 11 servings a day. They also recommended eating 2 to 4 servings of fruit (which is full of natural sugars) a day. These guidelines, even decades later, have been used as a framework for the US consumer education messages by the surgeon general, CDC, and many other government organizations since then.

Today, the ADA promotes eating "healthy carbohydrates" for diabetics instead of greatly reducing carbs from the diet. If carbs are ultimately sugar, and sugar ultimately causes many of these diseases, why are you told to prioritize carbs in your diet? There's no such thing as an essential carbohydrate. Your body can create the glucose it needs through a process called gluconeogenesis, where the liver converts glycerol (derived from fats) into glucose.

Alternatively, you've no doubt been taught that saturated and monounsaturated fats cause heart disease, cholesterol problems, and many other issues. In the last decade, dozens of studies and multiple meta-studies (studies that analyze other studies' results) with over 900,000 subjects from almost 100 different data sets have shown similar conclusions: Eating saturated and monounsaturated fats has no effects on heart disease risks, short- or long-term.

Most fats are good and are essential to our health—that's why there are *essential* fatty acids and *essential* amino acids (protein). Fats are the most efficient form of energy and each gram contains about 9 calories. That's more than double the amount in carbohydrates and protein (both have 4 calories per gram).

When you eat lots of fat and protein and greatly reduce carbs, your body adapts and converts the fat and protein, as well as the fat you have stored, into ketone bodies, or ketones, for energy. This metabolic process is called ketosis. That's where the *ketogenic* in ketogenic diet originates from.

This book will provide you with what you need to succeed with the ketogenic diet—simple cooking, weight loss, and long-term success.

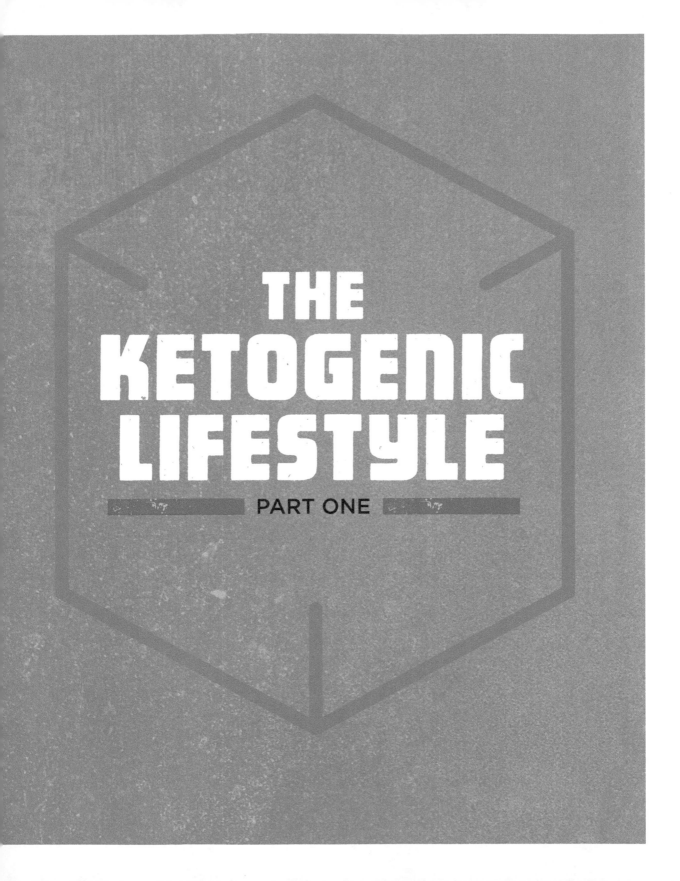

THE KETOGENIC LIFESTYLE

PART ONE

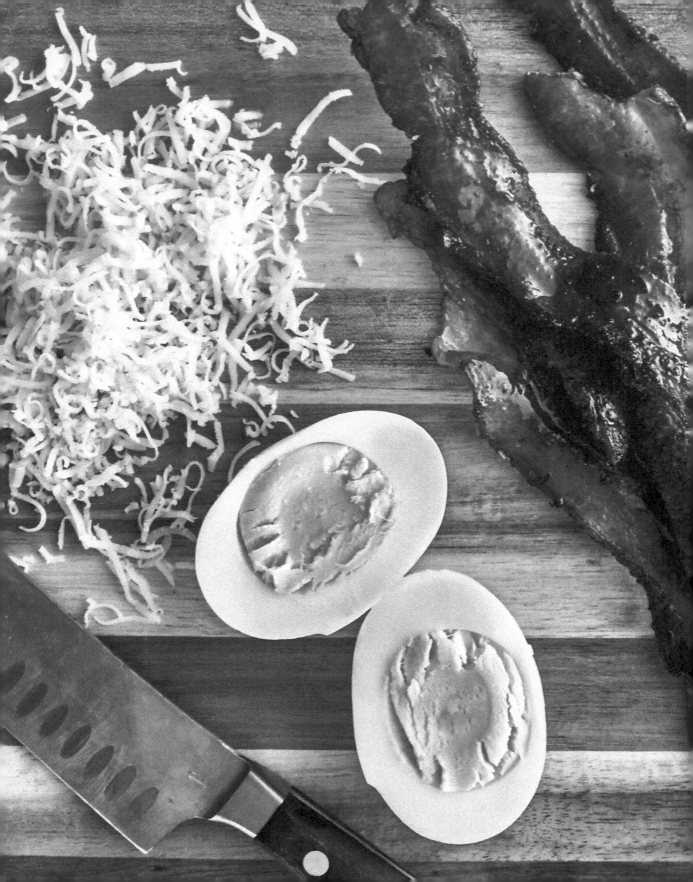

CHAPTER 1
LOW-CARB, HIGH-FAT

MAINTAINING A LOW-CARB, HIGH-FAT DIET is beneficial for weight loss. Most importantly, according to an increasing number of studies, it helps reduce risk factors for diabetes, heart diseases, stroke, Alzheimer's, epilepsy, and more. The keto diet promotes fresh whole foods like meat, fish, veggies, and healthy fats and oils, and greatly reduces processed, chemically treated foods. It's a diet that you can sustain long-term and enjoy. What's not to enjoy about a diet that encourages eating bacon and eggs for breakfast!

Carbs (sugar) cause blood glucose spikes, which result in crashes soon after, followed by cravings for more carbs. This cycle causes constant spikes in insulin and eventually may lead to prediabetes and type 2 diabetes.

Studies consistently show that a keto diet helps people lose more weight, improve energy levels throughout the day, and stay satiated longer. The increased satiety and improved energy levels are attributed to most of the calories coming from fat, which is very slow to digest and calorically dense. As a result, keto dieters commonly consume fewer calories because they're satiated longer and don't feel the need to eat as much or as often.

Why Go Keto?

When you eat a ketogenic diet, your body becomes efficient at burning fat for fuel. This is great for a multitude of reasons, not the least of which is that fat contains more than double the calories of most carbs, so you need to eat far less food by weight every day. Your body more readily burns the fat it has stored (the fat you're trying to get rid of), resulting in more weight loss. Using fat for fuel provides consistent energy levels, and it does not spike your blood glucose, so you don't experience the highs and lows when eating large amounts of carbs. Consistent energy levels throughout your day means you can get more done and feel less tired doing so.

In addition to those benefits, eating a keto diet in the long term has been proven to:

- Result in more weight loss (specifically body fat)
- Reduce blood sugar and insulin resistance (commonly reversing prediabetes and type 2 diabetes)
- Reduce triglyceride levels
- Reduce blood pressure
- Improve levels of HDL (good) and LDL (bad) cholesterol
- Improve brain function

Getting into Ketosis

When eating a high-carb diet, your body is in a metabolic state of glycolysis, which simply means that most of the energy your body uses comes from blood glucose. In this state, after each meal, your blood glucose is spiked causing higher levels of insulin, which promotes storage of body fat, and blocking the release of fat from your adipose (fat storage) tissues.

In contrast, a low-carb, high-fat diet puts your body into a metabolic state called ketosis. Your body breaks down fat into ketone bodies (ketones) for fuel as

SUPPORT FOR YOUR NEW LIFESTYLE

When starting the keto diet, it's important to let your closest friends and family members know you're serious about it and which foods you're trying to avoid. This will help during gatherings or outings. You may face some resistance in the beginning, and that's absolutely normal. The high-carb, low-fat diet has been the standard in most people's lives, and keto is a complete turnaround. Just focus on yourself and your progress. Soon enough, your high energy, weight loss, and overall positive outlook will make even naysayers curious.

A great place for initial support is reddit.com's keto subreddit: www.reddit.com/r/keto. You'll find hundreds of thousands of other keto-ers from around the world posting their experiences and progress, and supporting each other throughout their journeys.

its primary source of energy. In ketosis, your body readily burns fat for energy, and fat reserves are constantly released and consumed. It's a normal state—whenever you're low on carbs for a few days, your body will do this naturally.

Fats (fatty acids) and protein (amino acids) are essential for survival. There is no such thing as an essential carbohydrate. It simply does not exist.

Most cells in your body use ketones and glucose for fuel. For cells that can only take glucose, like parts of the brain, the glycerol derived from dietary fats is made into glucose by the liver through gluconeogenesis.

The main goal of the keto diet is to keep you in nutritional ketosis all the time. For those just starting the keto diet, to be fully keto-adapted usually takes anywhere from four to eight weeks.

Once you become keto-adapted, glycogen (the glucose stored in your muscles and liver) decreases, you carry less water weight, your muscle endurance increases, and your overall energy levels are higher than before. Also, if you kick yourself out of ketosis by eating too many carbs, you return to ketosis much sooner than when you were not keto-adapted. Additionally, once you are keto-adapted, you can generally eat up to 50 grams of carbs per day and still maintain ketosis.

WHAT TO DO IF YOU HAVE DIABETES

If you have diabetes, a low-carb diet can still work for you. For type 2 diabetes, it can begin to reverse the condition; for type 1 diabetics, it can greatly improve blood sugar control.

Always consult with your doctor before beginning a low-carb diet, especially with type 1 diabetes, because if you take medications, you may have to immediately decrease your doses. Your doctor may recommend doing a trial under their supervision so they can monitor your blood glucose levels and insulin doses. Additionally, for type 1 diabetes, you should eat over 50 grams of carbohydrates per day to prevent ketoacidosis.

Ketoacidosis is a toxic metabolic state that occurs when the body fails to regulate ketone production. The result is a severe accumulation of keto acids, which causes the pH of the blood to decrease substantially, making the blood more acidic. The most common causes for ketoacidosis are type 1 diabetes, prolonged alcoholism, and extreme starvation, which can result in diabetic ketoacidosis

The chart below provides the carbohydrate contents of commonly eaten foods for reference (fats, fish, poultry, and meats don't contain carbs):

FOOD	SERVING SIZE	CARBS (GRAMS)	CALORIES
POTATO	1 large, baked, plain	56	283
RICE	1 cup, white or brown	50	223
OATMEAL	1 cup, dry	49	339
PINTO BEANS (COOKED)	1 cup	45	245
BAGEL	1 whole	44	245
YOGURT	1 cup, fruit-flavored, low-fat	42	225
CORN (COOKED)	1 cup	41	177
SPAGHETTI	1 cup	40	221
PIZZA	1 slice, cheese	39	290
APPLE JUICE	1 cup	28	113
SWEET POTATO	1 large	28	118
ORANGE JUICE	1 cup	26	112
ENGLISH MUFFIN	1 whole	25	130
WAFFLE	1 (7-inch diameter)	25	218
BANANA	1 medium	24	105

FOOD	SERVING SIZE	CARBS (GRAMS)	CALORIES
APPLE	1 medium	21	81
CEREAL, READY TO EAT	1 cup	18	103
PANCAKE	1 (5-inch diameter)	15	90
MILK	1 cup	12	103
BREAD	1 slice, white	12	66
GREEN PEAS	½ cup	12	63
STRAWBERRIES	1 cup	11	45
CUCUMBER	1 (8-inch length)	9	47
YELLOW ONION	1 medium	8	44
BROCCOLI	1 stalk	6	51
ZUCCHINI	1 medium	4	33
CARROT	1 medium	4	25
TOMATO	1 medium	3	22
WHITE MUSHROOMS	1 cup	2	15
EGG	1 large	0.6	78
SPINACH	1 cup	0.4	7

(DKA), alcoholic ketoacidosis, and starvation ketoacidosis, respectively. Ketoacidosis rarely occurs for reasons other than type 1 diabetics.

Living in Ratios

Just like the USDA's Food Pyramid, the keto diet is built on ratios. It's important to get the right balance of macronutrients so your body has the energy it needs and you're not missing any essential fat or protein in your diet.

TESTING FOR KETOSIS

When you first start the keto diet, it's important to know if and when you're in ketosis when you first start eating low-carb. Not only is it a great confidence booster, but testing also lets you know that you're doing things right, or wrong, and whether you need to make any changes.

An easy test is to sniff for "keto-breath." After a few days, you might notice a taste that's somewhat fruity and a bit sour or even metallic. The reason for this? When your body is in ketosis, it creates the ketone bodies: acetone, acetoacetate, and beta-hydroxybutyrate. Acetone in particular is excreted through your urine and breath, which causes "keto-breath." This change in the smell of your breath and the taste in your mouth usually diminishes after a few weeks.

A more accurate way to tell is by using ketone urine test strips. They're fairly inexpensive and can instantly check the ketone levels in your urine. You can find them in packs of 100 for under $10 online or at most pharmacies. Try to take the test a few hours *after* you wake up in the morning, because being dehydrated after a night's sleep can cause a false positive.

The most accurate test involves a blood ketone meter. This type of test is a bit pricier at around $40 for the meter and up to $5 per test strip. The upside is it's much more accurate because it tests your blood directly. For nutritional ketosis, your reading should be between 0.5 and 5.0 millimeters.

Long term, it's not necessary to continuously check on your ketone levels. Within a few weeks, you'll know if you're eating right, and it becomes very easy to stay in ketosis.

Macronutrients are what foods are made of. They are fat, protein and carbo-hydrates. Each type of macronutrient provides a certain amount of energy (calories) per gram consumed.

- Fat provides about 9 calories per gram
- Protein provides about 4 calories per gram
- Carbohydrates provide about 4 calories per gram

On the keto diet, 65 to 75 percent of the calories you consume should come from fat. About 20 to 25 percent should come from protein, and the remaining 5 percent or so from carbohydrates.

Here are the same numbers broken down into an average 2000-calorie daily diet by grams and percentages:

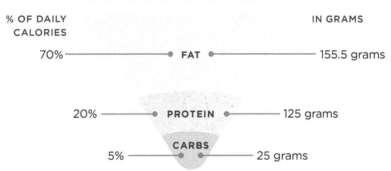

2000-CALORIE DAILY KETOGENIC DIET

% OF DAILY CALORIES		IN GRAMS
70%	FAT	155.5 grams
20%	PROTEIN	125 grams
5%	CARBS	25 grams

Keep in mind that 2000 calories is just an example—the number of calories you consume daily should be tailored to your body, activity levels, and goals.

The number of calories you should eat depends on a few factors, including:

- Current lean body weight (total body weight minus body fat)
- Daily activity levels (do you work in an office, wait tables, compete as a professional athlete?)
- Workout regimen? If so:
  - The types of workouts (weight lifting, cardio, or both)
  - Hours per week of each type

- Goal:
  - Lose weight
  - Maintain weight
  - Gain muscle

There are many ketogenic-based macro calculators available online, such as tasteaholics.com/keto-calculator and ketogains.com/ketogains-calculator. You can also find plenty of others through a quick Google search for "keto calculator." You'll be able to easily and quickly plug in your numbers and get an immediate estimation of your body's caloric needs.

One of the great things about the keto diet is that it's not necessary to track each and every number to hit your goals. Yet if you want to track, it's a great way to speed up your progress, and tracking will give you a visual reminder to stay on course every day.

Necessary Nutrients

It's crucial to drink plenty of water when beginning the keto diet. You may even notice that you're visiting the bathroom more often, and that's normal!

This happens because you're cutting out a lot of processed foods and have started eating more whole, natural foods instead. Processed foods have a lot of added sodium, and the sudden change in diet causes a sudden drop in sodium intake.

Additionally, the reduction in carbs reduces insulin levels, which in turn tells your kidneys to release excess stored sodium. Between the reduction in sodium intake and flushing of excess stored sodium, the body begins to excrete much more water than usual, and you end up low on sodium and other electrolytes.

When this happens, you may experience symptoms such as fatigue, headaches, coughing, sniffles, irritability, and/or nausea.

This state is generally known as the "keto flu." It's very important to know that this is not the actual influenza virus. It's called the keto flu only due to the similarity in symptoms, but it's neither contagious nor a real virus.

Many who experience these symptoms believe the keto diet made them sick and immediately go back to eating carbs. But the keto flu phase actually means your body is withdrawing from sugar, high carbs, and processed foods, and is readjusting so it can use fat as its fuel. The keto flu usually lasts just a few days while the body readjusts. You can abate its symptoms by adding more sodium and electrolytes to your diet.

Getting Ready to Go Keto

Now that you understand the benefits and science behind the ketogenic diet, you're ready to get started. In the following chapters, you'll get all the information you need to succeed with your keto diet, including what to buy and what to avoid, meal plans and full recipes, and how to exercise to maximize your health.

THE "KETO FLU"

The keto flu is avoidable and its duration can be reduced simply by adding more sodium to your diet. Here are some of the easiest ways to do it:

- Add more salt to your meals.
- Drink soup broths like beef and chicken.
- Eat saltier foods like pickled vegetables and bacon.

To replace other electrolytes, try to eat more of the foods listed below:

ELECTROLYTE	FOODS CONTAINING ELECTROLYTE
POTASSIUM	Avocados, nuts, dark leafy greens such as spinach and kale, salmon, plain yogurt, mushrooms
MAGNESIUM	Nuts, dark chocolate, artichokes, spinach, fish
CALCIUM	Cheeses, leafy greens, broccoli, seafood, almonds
PHOSPHORUS	Meats, cheeses, nuts, seeds, dark chocolate
CHLORIDE	Most vegetables, olives, salt, seaweed

Remember that if you don't feel better right away, it will pass within a couple of days, and you'll emerge a fat-burning machine!

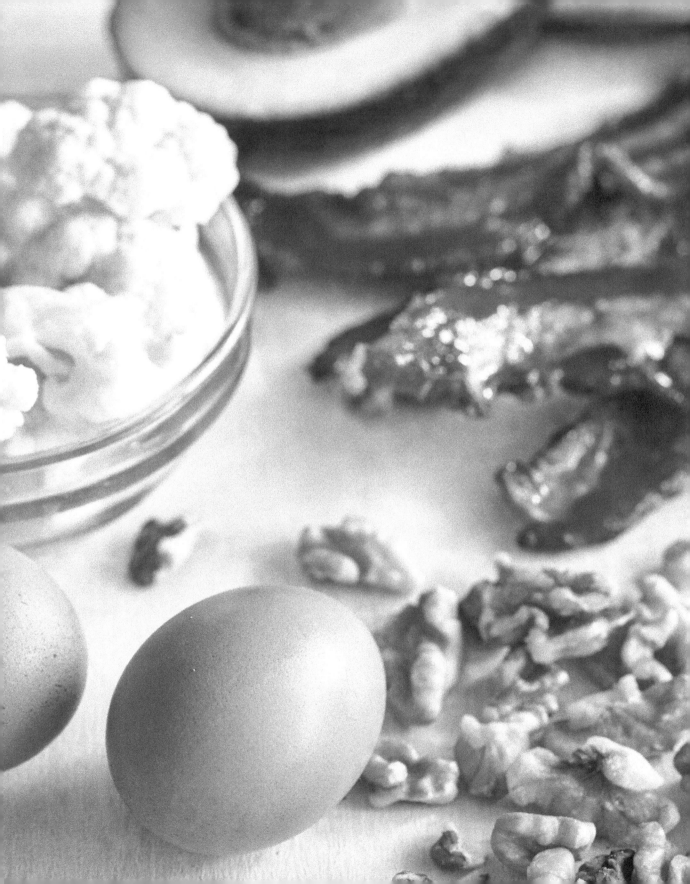

CHAPTER 2
GO KETO IN FIVE STEPS

YOU NOW KNOW THE SCIENCE behind the keto diet and why it works. In this chapter, you'll learn how to get started and maximize success. Here's a quick and easy step-by-step guide to use as you begin, and to refer to any time throughout your journey, for support and guidance.

Step 1: Clean Out Your Pantry

Out with the old, in with the new. Having tempting, unhealthy foods in your home is one of the biggest contributors to failure when starting any diet. To succeed, you need to minimize any triggers to maximize your chances. Unless you have the iron will of Arnold Schwarzenegger, you should not keep addictive foods like bread, desserts, and other non–keto friendly snacks around.

If you don't live alone, be sure to discuss and warn your housemates, whether they're significant others, family, or roommates. If some items must be kept (if they're simply not yours to throw out), try to agree on a special location to keep them out of sight. This will also help anyone you share your living space with understand that you are serious about starting your diet, and will lead to a better experience for you at home overall (people love to tempt anyone on a diet at first, but it will get old and they'll tire quickly).

STARCHES AND GRAINS

Get rid of all cereal, pasta, rice, potatoes, corn, oats, quinoa, flour, bread, bagels, wraps, rolls, and croissants.

SUGARY FOODS AND DRINKS

Get rid of all refined sugar, fountain drinks, fruit juices, milk, desserts, pastries, milk chocolate, candy bars, etc.

LEGUMES

Get rid of beans, peas, and lentils. They are dense with carbs. A 1-cup serving of beans alone contains more than three times the amount of carbs you want to consume in a day.

PROCESSED POLYUNSATURATED FATS AND OILS

Get rid of all vegetable oils and most seed oils, including sunflower, safflower, canola, soybean, grapeseed, and corn oil. Also eliminate trans fats like shortening and margarine—anything that says "hydrogenated" or "partially hydrogenated." Olive oil, extra-virgin olive oil, avocado oil, and coconut oil are the keto-friendly oils you want on hand.

FINDING SUPPORT

Sticking to your diet in the beginning can prove difficult when close friends and family aren't eating the same as you. Even worse, they are eating all the things you're trying not to eat. Every person is different, and you likely know who will support you and who will not. For those who support you, explain that you're avoiding carbs (and which foods include carbs) and request politely that they not offer you anything when you're eating together.

Telling the naysayers that you've quit eating grains and sugar will usually suffice. The terms *keto* and *low-carb* will usually spark a debate or argument with certain people because they've been told their whole lives to eat carbs and low-fat products. Try to avoid using those terms when explaining your diet goals. Avoid direct debates by recommending they read about the benefits of being in ketosis and the health benefits of eating a low-carb diet.

FRUITS

Get rid of fruits that are high in carbs, including bananas, dates, grapes, mangos, and apples. Be sure to get rid of any dried fruits like raisins as well. Dried fruit contains as much sugar as regular fruit but more concentrated, making it easy to eat a lot of sugar in a small serving. For comparison, a cup of raisins has over 100 grams of carbs while a cup of grapes has only 15 grams of carbs.

Yes, you're "getting rid" of unwanted foods in your pantry, but these foods can feed many others. Please, don't throw them away! Find a local food bank or homeless youth shelter to donate them to.

Your pantry will seem empty after the cleanout. That's because products meant for longer-term storage are usually high in carbs and full of unhealthy additives and preservatives. You'll fill your refrigerator shortly (Step 2) with healthy, natural foods.

Step 2: Go Shopping

It's time to restock your pantry, refrigerator, and freezer with delicious, keto-friendly foods that will help you lose weight, become healthy, and feel great!

THE BASICS

With these basics on hand, you'll always be ready to prepare healthy, delicious, and keto-friendly meals and snacks.

- Water, coffee, and tea
- All spices and herbs
- Sweeteners, including stevia and erythritol
- Lemon or lime juice
- Low-carb condiments like mayonnaise, mustard, pesto, and sriracha
- Broths (chicken, beef, bone)
- Pickled and fermented foods like pickles, kimchi, and sauerkraut
- Nuts and seeds, including macadamia nuts, pecans, almonds, walnuts, hazelnuts, pine nuts, flaxseed, chia seeds, and pumpkin seeds.

MEATS

Any type of meat is fine for the keto diet, including chicken, beef, lamb, pork, turkey, game, etc. It's preferable to use grass-fed and/or organic meats if they're available and possible for your budget. You can and should eat the fat on the meat and skin on the chicken.

All wild-caught fish and seafood slide into the keto diet nicely. Try to avoid farmed fish.

Go crazy with the eggs! Use organic eggs from free-range chickens, if possible.

VEGGIES

You can eat all nonstarchy veggies, including broccoli, asparagus, mushrooms, cucumbers, lettuce, onions, peppers, tomatoes, garlic (in small quantities—each clove contains about 1 gram of carbs), Brussels sprouts, eggplant, olives, zucchini, yellow squash, and cauliflower.

Avoid all types of potatoes, yams and sweet potatoes, corn, and legumes like beans, lentils, and peas.

ABOUT THOSE SWEETENERS . . .

The sweeteners may sound strange if you haven't heard of them before. They both come from natural sources and are safe to use in any quantity.

Stevia is extracted from the leaves of a plant called *Stevia rebaudiana*. Stevia has zero calories and contains some beneficial micronutrients like magnesium, potassium, and zinc. It's readily available in liquid or powder form online and in most supermarkets. It's much sweeter than sugar, so containers are usually very small—you won't need nearly as much.

Erythritol is a sugar alcohol that is low in calories, about 70 percent as sweet as sugar, and can be found naturally in some fruits and vegetables. Sugar alcohols are indigestible by the human body, so erythritol cannot raise your blood sugar or insulin levels. Several studies have proven it to be safe. Sugar alcohols can sometimes cause temporary digestive discomfort, but out of the few available sugar alcohols like xylitol, maltitol, and sorbitol, erythritol is considered to be the most forgiving and best for everyday use.

FRUITS

You can eat a small amount of berries every day, such as strawberries, raspberries, blackberries, and blueberries. Lemon and lime juices are great for adding flavor to your meals. Avocados are also low in carbs and full of healthy fat.

Avoid other fruits, as they're loaded with sugar. A single banana can contain around 25 grams of net carbs.

DAIRY

Eat full-fat dairy like butter, sour cream, heavy (whipping) cream, cheese, cream cheese, and unsweetened yogurt. Although not technically dairy, unsweetened almond and coconut milks are great as well.

Avoid milk and skim milk, as well as sweetened yogurt, as it contains a lot of sugar. Avoid any flavored, low-fat, or fat-free dairy products.

FATS AND OILS

Avocado oil, olive oil, butter, lard, and bacon fat are great for cooking and consuming. Avocado oil has a high smoke point (it does not burn or smoke until it reaches 520°F), which is ideal for searing meats and frying in a wok. Make sure to avoid oils labeled "blend"; they commonly contain small amounts of the healthy oil and large amounts of unhealthy oils.

Step 3: Set Up Your Kitchen

Preparing delicious recipes is one of the best parts of the keto diet, and it's quite easy if you have the right tools. The following tools will make cooking simpler and faster. Each one is worth investing in, especially for the busy cook.

FOOD SCALE

When you're trying to hit your caloric and macronutrient goals, a kitchen food scale is a necessary appliance. You can measure any solid or liquid food, and get the perfect amount every time. Used in combination with an app like MyFitnessPal, you'll have all the data you need to hit your goals sooner. Food scales can be found online for $10 to $20.

FOOD PROCESSOR

Food processors are critical to your arsenal. They are ideal for blending certain foods or processing foods together into sauces and shakes. Blenders don't cut it, powerwise, for many foods, especially tough vegetables like cauliflower.

One great food processor/blender is NutriBullet. The containers you blend in come with lids or drink spouts so you can take them to go or use them as storage. They're also easy to clean, making the whole system extremely convenient. They typically sell for about $80 online.

SPIRALIZER

Spiralizers make vegetables into noodles or ribbons within seconds. They make cooking a lot faster and easier—noodles have much more surface area and take a fraction of the time to cook. For example, a spiralizer turns a zucchini into zoodles, and with some Alfredo or marinara sauce, you can't tell you aren't eating noodles. Spiralizers cost around $30 and can be found in large retail stores and online.

ELECTRIC HAND MIXER

If you've ever had to beat an egg white by hand until you get stiff peaks, then you know just how difficult it is. Electric hand mixers save your arm muscles and massive amounts of time, especially when mixing heavy ingredients. You can find a decent one online for $10 to $20.

CAST IRON PANS

They've been used for centuries and were one of the first modern cooking devices. Cast iron skillets don't wear out and are healthier to use (no chemical treatment of any kind), retain heat very well, and can be moved between the stove and oven. They are simple to clean up—just wash them out with a scrub sponge without soap, dry them off, and then rub them with cooking oil. This prevents rust and encourages the buildup of "seasoning," a natural nonstick surface. Many cast iron pans come preseasoned, and this method preserves the coating. You can find them in many retail stores and online for $10 to $80, depending on the brand and size; Lodge is a popular brand, still made in the United States.

KETO-FRIENDLY ALTERNATIVES

You'd be surprised just how many carbs are in common everyday foods. Below is a chart of common foods and their keto-friendly alternatives that you can enjoy at any time.

Note: Net carbs are the total carbs minus dietary fiber (soluble and insoluble) and sugar alcohols. Fiber and sugar alcohols are not counted toward net carbs because the human body cannot digest and break them down into glucose, so they do not spike blood sugar.

NOT SO FRIENDLY	NET CARBS	QUANTITY	KETO-FRIENDLY ALTERNATIVE	NET CARBS
Milk	13 grams	1 cup	Unsweetened almond milk	0 grams
Pasta	41 grams	1 cup	Zucchini noodles	3 grams
Wraps or tortillas	18 grams	1 medium	Low-carb tortillas	6 grams
Sugar	25 grams	2 tablespoons	Stevia or erythritol	0 grams
Rice	44 grams	1 cup	Shirataki rice	0 grams
Mashed potatoes	22 grams	½ cup	Mashed cauliflower	4 grams
Bread crumbs	36 grams	½ cup	Almond flour	6 grams
Soda	39 grams	12 ounces	Water, tea, or coffee	0 grams
French fries	44 grams	4 ounces	Zucchini fries	3 grams
Potato chips	46 grams	3½ ounces	Mixed nuts	14 grams

NICE-TO-HAVE EQUIPMENT

The kitchen section of any store can be a wonderland. There are so many intriguing gadgets. It's also nice (although not necessary) to have these other tools on hand if you can't resist the lure:

INSTANT COOKING THERMOMETER Cooking steak and chicken is much easier when you can easily prod the meat and find out whether it's at the level of doneness that you're shooting for. These can usually be found for $10 to $20 in most retail stores or online.

MEASURING SPOON SET Get the right amount of an ingredient quickly. These sets can go from $5 to $10 in any supermarket, store, or online.

TONGS Tongs reduce splatter when working quickly (compared to using a fork or spatula to flip something in a hot pan). It's best to get tongs with nylon heads so you don't scratch any of your pots or pans. You can get a pair online or in retail stores for $10 to $15.

KNIFE SHARPENING STONE

Most of prep time is spent on cutting. You'll see your cutting speed skyrocket with a sharp knife set. It's also a pleasure to use sharp knives. Aim to sharpen your knives every week or so to keep them in good shape (professional chefs sharpen their knives before every use). Sharpening stones cost under $10 and can be ordered online.

Step 4: Meal Plan

Using meal plans in the beginning of your diet greatly increases your chances of success. The meal plans in part 2 of this book include meals for every part of the day, premade shopping lists, and macronutrient and calorie counts for each meal. They even account for leftovers. This will make starting out much easier and more enjoyable!

Meal plans work well because they give you goals and direction. If you know what you need to make next without thinking about it, you're less likely to give up, change your mind, and order food from your favorite takeout spot. Also, since you know what's coming next, you can look forward to it throughout the day and week.

After using the meal plans for a few weeks, you set your body up to have the right expectations for how much food you'll provide it and what type of food it will get (high in fat and protein and low in carbs). Even if you don't continue to use meal plans, you'll be familiar enough with the diet to know what you should be eating and how much.

Pay attention to the ingredients listed on the packaged products you buy. The best products have just a few ingredients with recognizable names, meaning they're made with fewer additives and preservatives.

CUSTOMIZING YOUR MEAL PLANS

Part 2 includes two weekly meal plans, which you can extend and reuse as many times as you like. You can also use the recipes from part 3 to make your own meal plans or swap out recipes in the meal plans provided.

The daily caloric goal in the meal plans is about 1700 calories, give or take 100 calories. If your caloric needs are higher or lower (don't forget to use an online keto calculator before you start), adjust accordingly with some of the ingredients in the meals by simply taking out a little or adding a bit more. Additionally, you can always use an extra tablespoon of olive oil or butter when cooking to get an extra 100 calories or so.

SHOPPING

Initially, you should look at the nutritional information provided for almost every packaged product to see if the product is low in carbs or not. Many companies love to add sugar, so be on the lookout. Over your first few weeks, you'll get to know which products are good and which are not as you look at nutritional labels.

Both of the meal plans in part 2 include shopping lists. You'll notice the quantities are not based on the quantities stores sell them in. Look for what would be closest to those amounts when buying the items. As you get more comfortable with your new diet and know the quantities you need, you'll rely less on shopping lists.

KETO QUOTIENT

All the recipes in this book are up to 6 grams of net carbs so you won't need to count the carbs when eating these recipes. Each recipe includes a Keto Quotient to make it easier to identify how high in fat it is.

KETO QUOTIENT	
GOOD	Up to 69 percent of the calories in the recipe come from fat
GREAT	70 to 79 percent of the calories in the recipe come from fat
EXCELLENT	80 percent or more of the calories in the recipe come from fat

Step 5: Exercise

As you start your diet and the pounds fall off, think about how to lose more weight or get healthier to feel even better. This is a great time to become more active through exercise.

Increase the amount you exercise relative to what you do now. If you don't exercise at all, start taking short walks or slow jogs, or a combination of both, for 15 minutes every other day. If you already go to the gym or lift weights, add an extra exercise or start doing cardio. It doesn't matter what level you're at, try to do a little more than you're doing now. That's all it takes to become healthier. Exercise is incremental, and every increment is a boost to weight loss and feeling better.

If you have the time, try taking a class or doing an activity that involves moving, like a step class or dancing, or start playing a sport like basketball. It doesn't have to be competitive, nor do you need to be good or have any previous experience. Such activities are an easy way to get on your feet, and you can learn a new skill in the process.

Staying fit through regular physical activity has been proven to reduce blood pressure and cholesterol levels as well as reduce risk for various heart diseases and type 2 diabetes. In combination with the keto diet, your health will improve dramatically, and so will your energy levels.

Any exercise, even if it's 15 minutes a week, is better than no exercise. Don't worry about how much you do in the beginning. Just start doing something and you'll build from there naturally.

EASY EXERCISE SEQUENCES

Here are a few easy exercise sequences if you're just starting out. Once every other day is enough in the beginning. If possible, try doing these with a friend or significant other for support and accountability. If you can't do some of them, that's absolutely all right! Simply focus on the ones you can do.

CARDIOVASCULAR ACTIVITY Any aerobic activity, like walking, running, or bicycling, for 15 to 30 minutes, twice a week or more.

STRENGTH CONDITIONING One set of exercises (for at least 10 repetitions, or it's too easy) targeting each of the major muscle groups: chest, shoulders, back, abs, and legs.
- Push-ups or assisted push-ups
- Pull-ups or chin-ups
- Crunches
- Squats

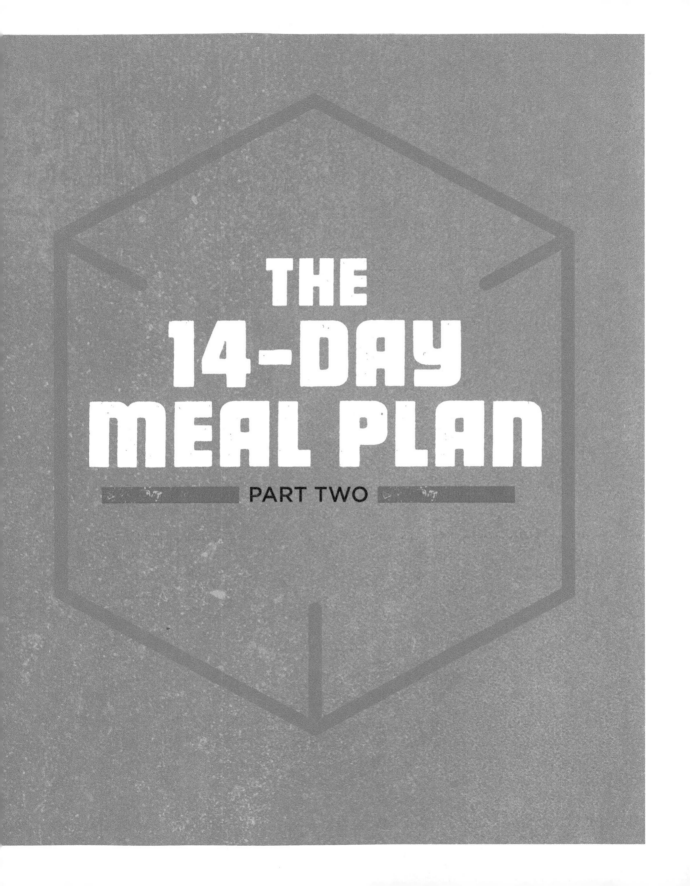

THE 14-DAY MEAL PLAN

PART TWO

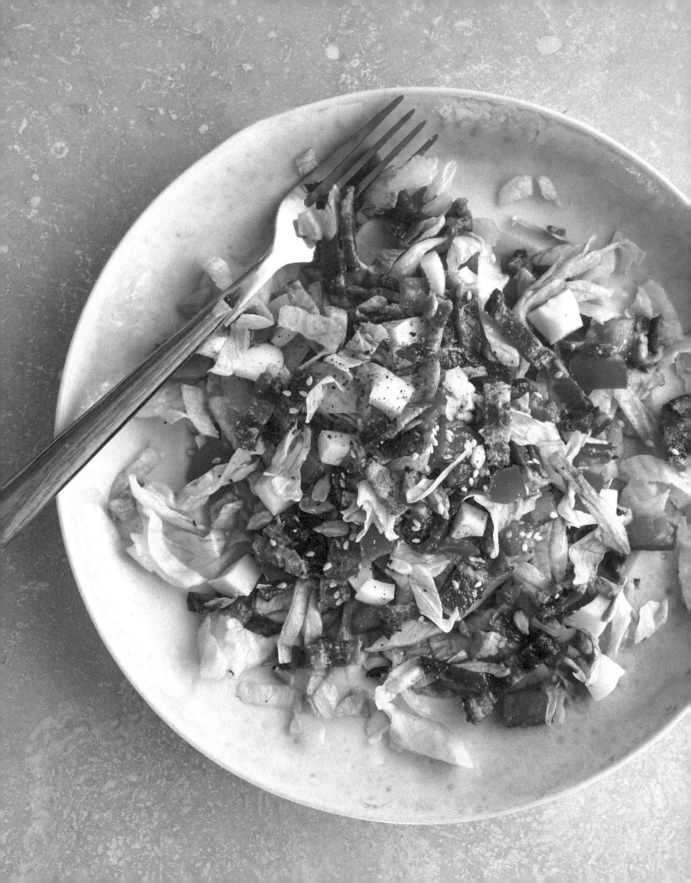

Week One and Week Two
Meal Plans and Shopping Lists

THE MEAL PLANS PROVIDED ON THE FOLLOWING PAGES are meant to give you a jump-start in your keto diet. Having a road map makes it easier to succeed, and besides, it's delicious.

Each day provides anywhere from 1600 to 1850 calories. If you don't know how many calories you should be eating, be sure to check out an online keto macro calculator. If you need to eat more calories than are provided in the meal plan, you can always add more of an ingredient or oil when you cook.

Please note: If you have any allergies or aversions to any of the ingredients, be sure to change them out for low-carb alternatives.

◀ BLT Salad, page 69

WEEK 1 MEAL PLAN

MONDAY

Breakfast: Nut Medley Granola (page 55)

Snack: Bacon-Cheese Deviled Eggs (2) (page 66)

Lunch: Chicken-Avocado Lettuce Wraps (page 70)

Snack: Creamy Cinnamon Smoothie (page 54)

Dinner: Lamb Leg with Sun-Dried Tomato Pesto (page 97) and Cheesy Mashed Cauliflower (page 111)

Per Day

Calories: 1840; Fat: 152g; Protein: 79g; Carbs: 39g; Fiber: 14g; Net Carbs: 25g

Fat 74% • Protein 20% • Carbs 6%

TUESDAY

Breakfast: Peanut Butter Cup Smoothie (page 50)

Snack: Walnut Herb-Crusted Goat Cheese (page 64)

Lunch: Cauliflower-Cheddar Soup (page 68)

Snack: Bacon-Cheese Deviled Eggs (2) (page 66)

Dinner: Lamb Leg with Sun-Dried Tomato Pesto (leftovers) (page 97) and Sautéed Crispy Zucchini (page 112)

Per Day

Calories: 1725; Fat: 139g; Protein: 87g; Carbs: 26g; Fiber: 10g; Net Carbs: 16g

Fat 74% • Protein 21% • Carbs 5%

WEDNESDAY

Breakfast: Avocado and Eggs (page 59)

Snack: Spinach-Blueberry Smoothie (page 53)

Lunch: Cauliflower Cheddar Soup (leftovers) (page 68)

Snack: Nutty Shortbread Cookies (page 124)

Dinner: Baked Coconut Haddock (page 81) and Brussels Sprouts Casserole (page 109)

Per Day

Calories: 1607; Fat: 123g; Protein: 77g; Carbs: 34g; Fiber: 17g; Net Carbs: 17g

Fat 77% • Protein 19% • Carbs 4%

THURSDAY

Breakfast: Lemon-Cashew Smoothie (page 52)

Snack: Almond Butter Fudge (2) (page 123)

Lunch: BLT Salad (page 69)

Snack: Bacon-Pepper Fat Bombs (page 62)

Dinner: Roasted Pork Loin with Grainy Mustard Sauce (page 93) and Golden Rosti (page 115)

Per Day

Calories: 1637; Fat: 137g; Protein: 79g; Carbs: 26g; Fiber: 6g; Net Carbs: 20g

Fat 75% • Protein 20% • Carbs 5%

FRIDAY

Breakfast: Berry Green Smoothie (page 51)

Snack: Bacon-Pepper Fat Bombs (2) (page 62)

Lunch: Roasted Pork Loin with Grainy Mustard Sauce (leftovers) (page 93)

Snack: Vanilla-Almond Ice Pops (page 125)

Dinner: Turkey Meatloaf (page 88) and Golden Rosti (page 115)

Per Day

Calories: 1635; Fat: 134g; Protein: 85g; Carbs: 21g; Fiber: 7g; Net Carbs: 14g

Fat 74% • Protein 21% • Carbs 5%

SATURDAY

Breakfast: Breakfast Bake (page 58)

Snack: Creamy Cinnamon Smoothie (page 54)

Lunch: Turkey Meatloaf (leftovers) (page 88)

Snack: Nutty Shortbread Cookies (page 124)

Dinner: Cheesy Garlic Salmon (page 82) and Garlicky Green Beans (page 107)

Per Day

Calories: 1633; Fat: 137g; Protein: 81g; Carbs: 19g; Fiber: 5g; Net Carbs: 14g

Fat 76% • Protein 20% • Carbs 4%

SUNDAY

Breakfast: Nut Medley Granola (page 55)

Snack: Smoked Salmon Fat Bombs (page 63)

Lunch: Breakfast Bake (page 58)

Snack: Almond Butter Fudge (2) (page 123)

Dinner: Chicken Bacon Burger (page 82) and Portobello Mushroom Pizza (page 106)

Per Day

Calories: 1712; Fat: 143g; Protein: 79g; Carbs: 27g; Fiber: 13g; Net Carbs: 14g

Fat 75% • Protein 20% • Carbs 5%

WEEK 1 SHOPPING LIST

MEAT AND SEAFOOD

Bacon (44 slices)

Chicken breast, boneless (6 ounces)

Chicken, ground (1 pound)

Haddock fillets, 4 boneless (5 ounces each)

Lamb leg (2 pounds)

Pork loin roast, boneless (2 pounds)

Salmon fillets, 4 boneless (5 ounces each)

Salmon, smoked (2 ounces)

Sausage, preservative-free or
   homemade (1 pound)

Turkey, ground (1½ pounds)

DAIRY, DAIRY ALTERNATIVES, AND EGGS

Almond milk (2 cups)

Asiago cheese (½ cup)

Butter (2 cups)

Cashew milk, unsweetened (1 cup)

Cheddar cheese, shredded (2¼ cups)

Coconut cream (¾ cup)

Coconut milk beverage (3 cups)

Cream cheese (5 ounces)

Eggs (20)

Goat cheese (12 ounces)

Heavy (whipping) cream (5⅓ cups)

Mozzarella cheese, shredded (1 cup)

Parmesan cheese (1 cup)

Swiss cheese (1¼ cups)

PRODUCE

Acorn squash (1)

Avocados (4)

Basil, fresh (1 bunch)

Blueberries (1 pint)

Boston lettuce (2 heads)

Brussels sprouts (1 pound)

Cauliflower (2)

Celeriac (1)

English cucumber (1)

Garlic cloves (12)

Green beans (1 pound)

Kale (2 ounces)

Lemons (2)

Mint sprigs, fresh (1 bunch)

Onion, sweet (1)

Oregano, fresh (1 bunch)

Parsley, fresh (1 bunch)

Portobello mushrooms (4)

Raspberries (1 pint)

Spaghetti squash (1)

Spinach (1 cup)

Thyme, fresh (1 bunch)

Tomato (2)

Zucchini (4)

CANNED AND BOTTLED ITEMS

Almond butter (2 cups)

Chicken stock (4 cups)

Coconut milk (2 cups)

Coconut oil (2 cups)

Dijon mustard (½ teaspoon)

Grainy mustard (3 tablespoons)

Mayonnaise (⅔ cup)

Olive oil (1 cup)

Olive oil, extra-virgin (2 tablespoons)

Red wine vinegar (2 tablespoons)

Stevia, liquid (30 drops)

Sun-dried tomatoes packed in oil (1 cup)

Vanilla extract, alcohol-free (2 teaspoons)

PANTRY ITEMS

Almonds, ground (1¾ cup)

Almonds, sliced (1 cup)

Black pepper, freshly ground

Cinnamon, ground (3 teaspoons)

Coconut, shredded unsweetened (4 cups)

Hazelnuts, ground (¾ cup)

Nutmeg, ground (1 teaspoon)

Peanut butter (2 tablespoons)

Pine nuts (¼ cup)

Protein powder, chocolate (2 tablespoons)

Protein powder, plain (4 tablespoons)

Protein powder, vanilla (8 tablespoons)

Pumpkin seeds, raw (½ cup)

Sea salt

Sesame seeds (1 teaspoon)

Sunflower seeds, raw (1¼ cups)

Sweetener, granulated (⅔ cup)

Vanilla bean (2)

Walnuts, chopped (10 ounces)

WEEK 2 MEAL PLAN

MONDAY

Breakfast: Berry Green Smoothie (page 51)

Snack: Nutty Shortbread Cookies (page 124)

Lunch: Chicken-Avocado Lettuce Wraps (page 70)

Snack: Crispy Parmesan Crackers (page 65)

Dinner: Baked Coconut Haddock (page 81) and Brussels Sprouts Casserole (page 109)

Per Day

Calories: 1622; Fat: 126g; Protein: 88g; Carbs: 34g; Fiber: 15g; Net Carbs: 19g

Fat 70% • Protein 22% • Carbs 8%

TUESDAY

Breakfast: Nut Medley Granola (page 55)

Snack: Vanilla-Almond Ice Pops (page 125)

Lunch: Crab Salad–Stuffed Avocado (page 71)

Snack: Chocolate-Coconut Treats (2) (page 122)

Dinner: Lamb Leg with Sun-Dried Tomato Pesto (page 97) and Brussels Sprouts Casserole (page 109)

Per Day

Calories: 1606; Fat: 130g; Protein: 77g; Carbs: 35g; Fiber: 17g; Net Carbs: 18g

Fat 73% • Protein 20% • Carbs 7%

WEDNESDAY

Breakfast: Peanut Butter Cup Smoothie (page 50)

Snack: Crispy Parmesan Crackers (page 65)

Lunch: BLT Salad (page 69)

Snack: Smoked Salmon Fat Bombs (page 63)

Dinner: Lamb Leg with Sun-Dried Tomato Pesto (leftovers) (page 97) and Cheesy Mashed Cauliflower (page 111)

Per Day

Calories: 1604; Fat: 130g; Protein: 86g; Carbs: 23g; Fiber: 9g; Net Carbs: 14g

Fat 73% • Protein 21% • Carbs 6%

THURSDAY

Breakfast: Avocado and Eggs (page 59)

Snack: Almond Butter Fudge (2) (page 123)

Lunch: Cauliflower-Cheddar Soup (page 68)

Snack: Berry Green Smoothie (page 51)

Dinner: Herb Butter Scallops (page 75) and Pesto Zucchini Noodles (page 114)

Per Day

Calories: 1720; Fat: 140g; Protein: 83g; Carbs: 32g; Fiber: 13g; Net Carbs: 19g

Fat 73% • Protein 20% • Carbs 7%

FRIDAY

Breakfast: Lemon-Cashew Smoothie (page 52)

Snack: Peanut Butter Mousse (page 127)

Lunch: Cauliflower-Cheddar Soup (leftovers) (page 68)

Snack: Chocolate-Coconut Treats (page 122)

Dinner: Roasted Pork Loin with Grainy Mustard Sauce (page 93) and Mushrooms with Camembert (page 113)

Per Day

Calories: 1707; Fat: 139g; Protein: 84g; Carbs: 30g; Fiber: 7g; Net Carbs: 23g

Fat 73% • Protein 20% • Carbs 7%

SATURDAY

Breakfast: Breakfast Bake (page 58)

Snack: Queso Dip (page 67)

Lunch: Roasted Pork Loin with Grainy Mustard Sauce (leftovers) (page 93)

Snack: Almond Butter Fudge (3) (page 123)

Dinner: Lemon Butter Chicken (page 83) and Sautéed Asparagus with Walnuts (page 108)

Per Day

Calories: 1651; Fat: 142g; Protein: 75g; Carbs: 20g; Fiber: 5g; Net Carbs: 14g

Fat 76% • Protein 20% • Carbs 4%

SUNDAY

Breakfast: Nut Medley Granola (page 55)

Snack: Chicken-Avocado Lettuce Wraps (page 70)

Lunch: Breakfast Bake (page 58)

Snack: Raspberry Cheesecake (page 126) with ¼ cup whipped cream*

Dinner: Turkey Meatloaf (page 88) and Creamed Spinach (page 110)

Per Day

Calories: 1697; Fat: 140g; Protein: 71g; Carbs: 31g; Fiber: 13g; Net Carbs: 18g

Fat 74% • Protein 20% • Carbs 6%

*Add a dollop of freshly whipped cream to your Raspberry Cheesecake

WEEK 2 SHOPPING LIST

MEAT AND SEAFOOD

Bacon (14 slices)

Chicken breast, 2 boneless (6 ounces each)

Chicken thighs, bone-in, skin-on (4)

Dungeness crab meat (4½ ounces)

Haddock fillets, 4 boneless (5 ounces each)

Lamb leg (2 pounds)

Pork loin roast, boneless (2 pounds)

Sausage, preservative-free
    or homemade (1 pound)

Sea scallops (1 pound)

Turkey, ground (1½ pounds)

DAIRY, DAIRY ALTERNATIVES, AND EGGS

Almond milk (2 cups)

Butter (1¼ cups)

Camembert cheese (4 ounces)

Cashew milk, unsweetened (1 cup)

Cheddar cheese (13 ounces)

Coconut cream (¾ cup)

Coconut milk beverage (½ cup)

Cream cheese (1¾ cups)

Eggs (20)

Goat cheese (2 ounces)

Heavy (whipping) cream (6⅓ cups)

Parmesan cheese (10 ounces)

Swiss cheese (4 ounces)

PRODUCE

Asparagus (¾ pound)

Avocados (4)

Basil, fresh (1 bunch)

Bell pepper, red (1)

Boston lettuce (2 heads)

Brussels sprouts (1 pound)

Button mushrooms (1 pound)

Cauliflower (2)

Cilantro (1 bunch)

English cucumber (1)

Garlic cloves (10)

Jalapeño pepper (1)

Kale (1 bunch)

Lemons (3)

Onions, sweet (2)

Oregano, fresh (1 bunch)

Parsley, fresh (1 bunch)

Raspberries (2 pints)

Scallion (1)

Spaghetti squash (1)

Spinach (3 ounces)

Thyme, fresh (1 bunch)

Tomato (1)

Zucchini (4)

CANNED AND BOTTLED ITEMS

Almond butter (2 cups)

Chicken stock (4¾ cups)

Coconut oil (1¾ cups)

Grainy mustard (3 tablespoons)

Mayonnaise (⅓ cup)

Olive oil (½ cup)

Olive oil, extra-virgin (6 tablespoons)

Red wine vinegar (2 tablespoons)

Stevia, liquid (18 drops)

Sun-dried tomatoes packed in oil (1 cup)

Vanilla extract, alcohol-free (2 teaspoons)

PANTRY ITEMS

Almond flour (1½ cups)

Almonds, sliced (1 cup)

Baking powder (½ teaspoon)

Black pepper, freshly ground

Cayenne pepper (¼ teaspoon)

Cinnamon, ground (1 teaspoon)

Cocoa powder (¼ cup)

Coconut, shredded unsweetened (3¼ cups)

Hazelnuts, ground (¼ cup)

Nutmeg, ground (1 teaspoon)

Nutritional yeast (2 teaspoons)

Onion powder (½ teaspoon)

Peanut butter (6 tablespoons)

Pine nuts (¼ cup)

Protein powder, chocolate (2 tablespoons)

Protein powder, plain (2 tablespoons)

Protein powder, vanilla (2 tablespoons)

Pumpkin seeds (½ cup)

Sea salt

Sesame seeds (1 teaspoon)

Sunflower seeds (1 cup)

Sweetener, granulated (¼ cup)

Walnuts, chopped (1 cup)

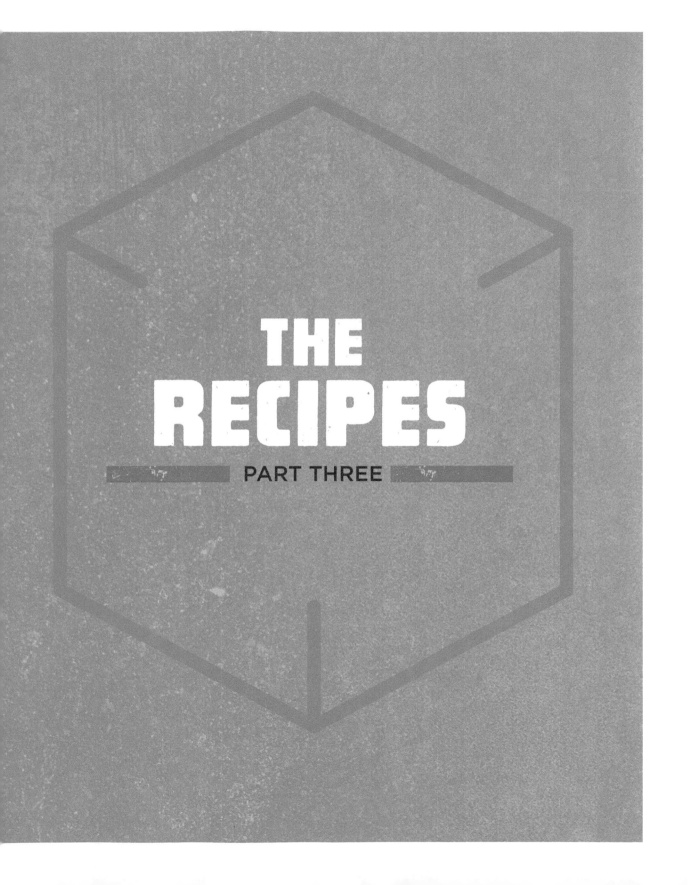

THE RECIPES

PART THREE

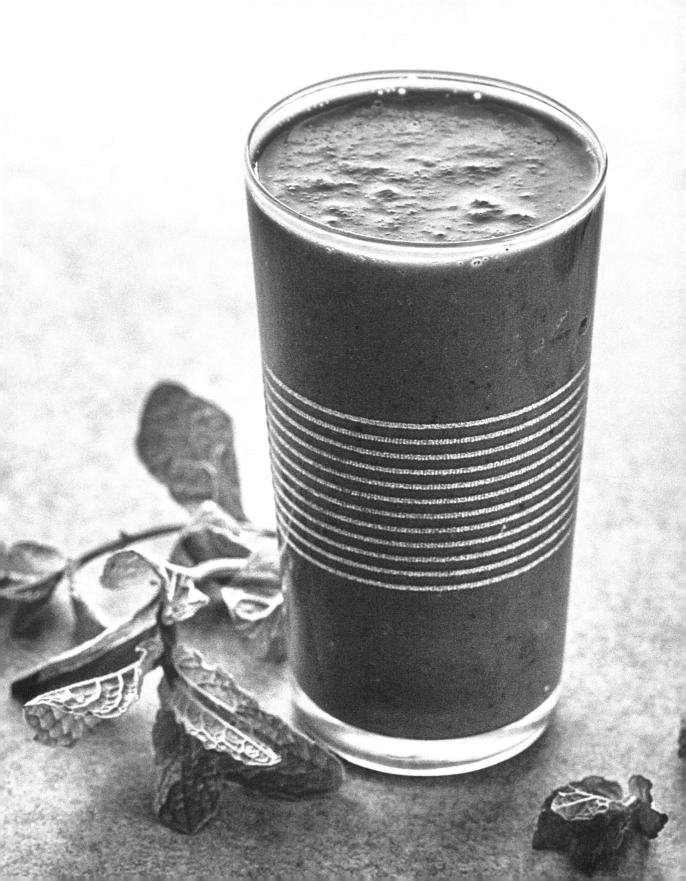

SMOOTHIES & BREAKFASTS

◄ Spinach-Blueberry Smoothie, page 53

PEANUT BUTTER CUP SMOOTHIE

Serves 2 / Prep time: 5 minutes

Lovers of the popular candy featuring chocolate and peanut butter will enjoy the same flavor combination for breakfast or a filling snack. For a more chocolaty taste, add a teaspoon of good-quality cocoa powder and a couple drops of liquid stevia. These additions will not add any fat, protein, or carbs to the smoothie, just 3 calories per serving.

1 cup water

¾ cup coconut cream

1 scoop chocolate protein powder

2 tablespoons natural peanut butter

3 ice cubes

1. Put the water, coconut cream, protein powder, peanut butter, and ice in a blender and blend until smooth.
2. Pour into 2 glasses and serve immediately.

PER SERVING Calories: 486; Fat: 40g; Protein: 30g; Carbs: 11g; Fiber: 5g; Net Carbs: 6g; Fat 70%/Protein 20%/Carbs 10%

BERRY GREEN SMOOTHIE

Serves 2 / Prep time: 10 minutes

You might be taken aback by the unusual color of this smoothie—it's kind of greenish brown—but the taste is similar to raspberry cheesecake. Kale is a perfect addition to smoothies because it has a less assertive taste than some other greens. Kale is also a spectacular source of vitamin K and very high in vitamins A and C.

1 cup water

½ cup raspberries

½ cup shredded kale

¾ cup cream cheese

1 tablespoon coconut oil

1 scoop vanilla protein powder

1. Put the water, raspberries, kale, cream cheese, coconut oil, and protein powder in a blender and blend until smooth.

2. Pour into 2 glasses and serve immediately.

PER SERVING Calories: 436; Fat: 36g; Protein: 28g; Carbs: 11g; Fiber: 5g; Net Carbs: 6g; Fat 70%/Protein 20%/Carbs 10%

LEMON-CASHEW SMOOTHIE

Serves 1 / Prep time: 5 minutes

The cashew milk and heavy cream combine to create an absolutely luscious smoothie that is tart enough to be refreshing and still makes for a satisfying breakfast or snack. If you add a few ice cubes, it will be like enjoying a rich citrus sorbet instead of a healthy breakfast. A couple leaves of fresh mint will also enhance the fresh flavor.

1 cup unsweetened cashew milk

¼ cup heavy (whipping) cream

¼ cup freshly squeezed lemon juice

1 scoop plain protein powder

1 tablespoon coconut oil

1 teaspoon sweetener

1. Put the cashew milk, heavy cream, lemon juice, protein powder, coconut oil, and sweetener in a blender and blend until smooth.
2. Pour into a glass and serve immediately.

SUBSTITUTION TIP Almond milk or coconut milk are also fine choices instead of cashew milk if you prefer those products. Each type of milk adds a slightly different flavor to the smoothie, so try them all to get the right combination for your palate.

PER SERVING Calories: 503; Fat: 45g; Protein: 29g; Carbs: 15g; Fiber: 4g; Net Carbs: 11g; Fat 80%/Protein 13%/Carbs 7%

SPINACH-BLUEBERRY SMOOTHIE

Serves 2 / Prep time: 5 minutes

NUT FREE
VEGETARIAN
UNDER 30 MINUTES

Blueberries are the second most popular berry in the United States and have one of the highest antioxidant contents of any food. Throwing a handful of this fruit in your morning smoothie adds vitamins K and C, magnesium, and copper to your diet. Look for organic berries because they have a higher antioxidant level than conventionally grown fruit.

1 cup coconut milk

1 cup spinach

½ English cucumber, chopped

½ cup blueberries

1 scoop plain protein powder

2 tablespoons coconut oil

4 ice cubes

Mint sprigs, for garnish

1. Put the coconut milk, spinach, cucumber, blueberries, protein powder, coconut oil, and ice in a blender and blend until smooth.

2. Pour into 2 glasses, garnish each with the mint, and serve immediately.

PER SERVING Calories: 353; Fat: 32g; Protein: 15g; Carbs: 9g; Fiber: 3g; Net Carbs: 6g; Fat 76%/Protein 16%/Carbs 8%

CREAMY CINNAMON SMOOTHIE

Serves 2 / Prep time: 5 minutes

Cinnamon is a lovely warm spice that often conjures up visions of holiday desserts or fragrant baked goods. Try to find Ceylon cinnamon instead of Cassia, because it does not contain cormarin, a toxin that affects the liver. Ceylon cinnamon is lighter in color and has a more delicate flavor than Cassia.

2 cups coconut milk
1 scoop vanilla protein powder
5 drops liquid stevia

1 teaspoon ground cinnamon
½ teaspoon alcohol-free
  vanilla extract

1. Put the coconut milk, protein powder, stevia, cinnamon, and vanilla in a blender and blend until smooth.
2. Pour into 2 glasses and serve immediately.

A CLOSER LOOK Most of the vanilla you will find in the grocery store probably has alcohol in it because vanilla extract in the United States cannot be called pure unless it is 35 percent alcohol. You can find vanilla extract without alcohol in specialty stores, or use imitation vanilla extract.

PER SERVING Calories: 492; Fat: 47g; Protein: 18g; Carbs: 8g; Fiber: 2g; Net Carbs: 6g; Fat 80%/Protein 14%/Carbs 6%

NUT MEDLEY GRANOLA

Serves 8 / Prep time: 10 minutes / Cook time: 1 hour

KETO QUOTIENT

DAIRY FREE
GLUTEN FREE
VEGETARIAN

Homemade granola is an incredibly versatile treat to have on hand for breakfast, snacks, and as a healthy topping for a creamy cup of Greek yogurt. The combination and amount of nuts in this recipe creates a wonderful keto macro, but you can add or omit different ingredients to suit your taste. Stay away from adding dried fruits though, because they are very high in carbs.

2 cups shredded unsweetened
  coconut
1 cup sliced almonds
1 cup raw sunflower seeds
½ cup raw pumpkin seeds

½ cup walnuts
½ cup melted coconut oil
10 drops liquid stevia
1 teaspoon ground cinnamon
½ teaspoon ground nutmeg

1. Preheat the oven to 250°F. Line 2 baking sheets with parchment paper. Set aside.

2. Toss together the shredded coconut, almonds, sunflower seeds, pumpkin seeds, and walnuts in a large bowl until mixed.

3. In a small bowl, stir together the coconut oil, stevia, cinnamon, and nutmeg until blended.

4. Pour the coconut oil mixture into the nut mixture and use your hands to blend until the nuts are very well coated.

5. Transfer the granola mixture to the baking sheets and spread it out evenly.

6. Bake the granola, stirring every 10 to 15 minutes, until the mixture is golden brown and crunchy, about 1 hour.

7. Transfer the granola to a large bowl and let the granola cool, tossing it frequently to break up the large pieces.

8. Store the granola in airtight containers in the refrigerator or freezer for up to 1 month.

PER SERVING Calories: 391; Fat: 38g; Protein: 10g; Carbs: 10g; Fiber: 6g;
Net Carbs: 4g; Fat 80%/Protein 10%/Carbs 10%

BACON-ARTICHOKE OMELET

Serves 4 / Prep time: 10 minutes / Cook time: 10 minutes

Omelets are not just for breakfast, and this vegetable- and bacon-packed beauty is hearty enough for a light dinner. If you add a nice mixed green salad to the plate, you won't go over your carbs because the combination with the omelet should still be an excellent keto macro. If you have leftovers, try them cold the next day for a snack or lunch.

6 eggs, beaten

2 tablespoons heavy (whipping) cream

8 bacon slices, cooked and chopped

1 tablespoon olive oil

¼ cup chopped onion

½ cup chopped artichoke hearts (canned, packed in water)

Sea salt

Freshly ground black pepper

1. In a small bowl, whisk together the eggs, heavy cream, and bacon until well blended, and set aside.

2. Place a large skillet over medium-high heat and add the olive oil.

3. Sauté the onion until tender, about 3 minutes.

4. Pour the egg mixture into the skillet, swirling it for 1 minute.

5. Cook the omelet, lifting the edges with a spatula to let the uncooked egg flow underneath, for 2 minutes.

6. Sprinkle the artichoke hearts on top and flip the omelet. Cook for 4 minutes more, until the egg is firm. Flip the omelet over again so the artichoke hearts are on top.

7. Remove from the heat, cut the omelet into quarters, and season with salt and black pepper. Transfer the omelet to plates and serve.

PER SERVING Calories: 435; Fat: 39g; Protein: 17g; Carbs: 5g; Fiber: 2g; Net Carbs: 3g; Fat 80%/Protein 15%/Carbs 5%

MUSHROOM FRITTATA

Serves 6 / Prep time: 10 minutes / Cook time: 15 minutes

KETO QUOTIENT

GLUTEN FREE
NUT FREE
UNDER 30 MINUTES

Frittatas can be described as baked omelets or as crustless quiches, but no matter what the description, they are delicious and simple. Any type of mushrooms can be used for the recipe depending on what you like or what you have in your refrigerator. If you want to use portobello mushrooms, scoop out the black gills so that your eggs don't turn an unsightly gray.

2 tablespoons olive oil
1 cup sliced fresh mushrooms
1 cup shredded spinach
6 bacon slices, cooked
   and chopped

10 large eggs, beaten
½ cup crumbled goat cheese
Sea salt
Freshly ground black pepper

1. Preheat the oven to 350°F.
2. Place a large ovenproof skillet over medium-high heat and add the olive oil.
3. Sauté the mushrooms until lightly browned, about 3 minutes.
4. Add the spinach and bacon and sauté until the greens are wilted, about 1 minute.
5. Add the eggs and cook, lifting the edges of the frittata with a spatula so uncooked egg flows underneath, for 3 to 4 minutes.
6. Sprinkle the top with the crumbled goat cheese and season lightly with salt and pepper.
7. Bake until set and lightly browned, about 15 minutes.
8. Remove the frittata from the oven, and let it stand for 5 minutes.
9. Cut into 6 wedges and serve immediately.

SUBSTITUTION TIP If you're not keen on goat cheese, feta cheese tastes lovely with the other ingredients in this dish. Feta is higher in fat and lower in protein than goat cheese, so keep that in mind when considering your keto macros.

PER SERVING Calories: 316; Fat: 27g; Protein: 16g; Carbs: 1g; Fiber: 0g; Net Carbs: 1g; Fat 80%/Protein 16%/Carbs 4%

BREAKFAST BAKE

Serves 8 / Prep time: 10 minutes / Cook time: 50 minutes

Spaghetti squash adds a satisfying texture and bulk to this casserole as well as a plethora of nutritional benefits. It is high in vitamins A, B, and C, which are powerful antioxidants. Spaghetti squash is also an excellent source of beta-carotene, potassium, manganese, and calcium.

1 tablespoon olive oil, plus extra
  for greasing the casserole dish
1 pound preservative-free
  or homemade sausage
8 large eggs
2 cups cooked spaghetti squash

1 tablespoon chopped
  fresh oregano
Sea salt
Freshly ground black pepper
½ cup shredded Cheddar cheese

1. Preheat the oven to 375°F. Lightly grease a 9-by-13-inch casserole dish with olive oil and set aside.

2. Place a large ovenproof skillet over medium-high heat and add the olive oil.

3. Brown the sausage until cooked through, about 5 minutes. While the sausage is cooking, whisk together the eggs, squash, and oregano in a medium bowl. Season lightly with salt and pepper and set aside.

4. Add the cooked sausage to the egg mixture, stir until just combined, and pour the mixture into the casserole dish.

5. Sprinkle the top of the casserole with the cheese and cover the casserole loosely with aluminum foil.

6. Bake the casserole for 30 minutes, and then remove the foil and bake for an additional 15 minutes.

7. Let the casserole stand for 10 minutes before serving.

PER SERVING Calories: 303; Fat: 24g; Protein: 17g; Carbs: 4g; Fiber: 1g;
Net Carbs: 3g; Fat 72%/Protein 23%/Carbs 5%

AVOCADO AND EGGS

Serves 4 / Prep time: 10 minutes / Cook time: 20 minutes

These pale green egg-filled fruits are a lovely light breakfast and the perfect keto macro to start the day. The avocados should be ripe but still firm so they hold together when baked. Avocados are very high in healthy fats, about 25 grams per cup, and are packed with antioxidants. The best way to peel an avocado is to nick the peel and remove it by hand. The greatest concentration of phytonutrients is in the darker flesh right next to the peel.

2 avocados, peeled, halved
   lengthwise, and pitted
4 large eggs
1 (4-ounce) chicken breast,
   cooked and shredded

¼ cup Cheddar cheese
Sea salt
Freshly ground black pepper

1. Preheat the oven to 425°F.
2. Take a spoon and hollow out each side of the avocado halves until the hole is about twice the original size.
3. Place the avocado halves in an 8-by-8-inch baking dish, hollow-side up.
4. Crack an egg into each hollow and divide the shredded chicken between each avocado half. Sprinkle the cheese on top of each and season lightly with the salt and pepper.
5. Bake the avocados until the eggs are cooked through, about 15 to 20 minutes.
6. Serve immediately.

PREP TIP Cooked chicken breast is very handy for many recipes, so bake 4 or 5 breasts at the beginning of the week and store them in a sealed plastic bag in the refrigerator after they are completely cooled. Cooked chicken will keep for up to 5 days in the refrigerator.

PER SERVING Calories: 324; Fat: 25g; Protein: 19g; Carbs: 8g; Fiber: 5g; Net Carbs: 3g; Fat 70%/Protein 20%/Carbs 10%

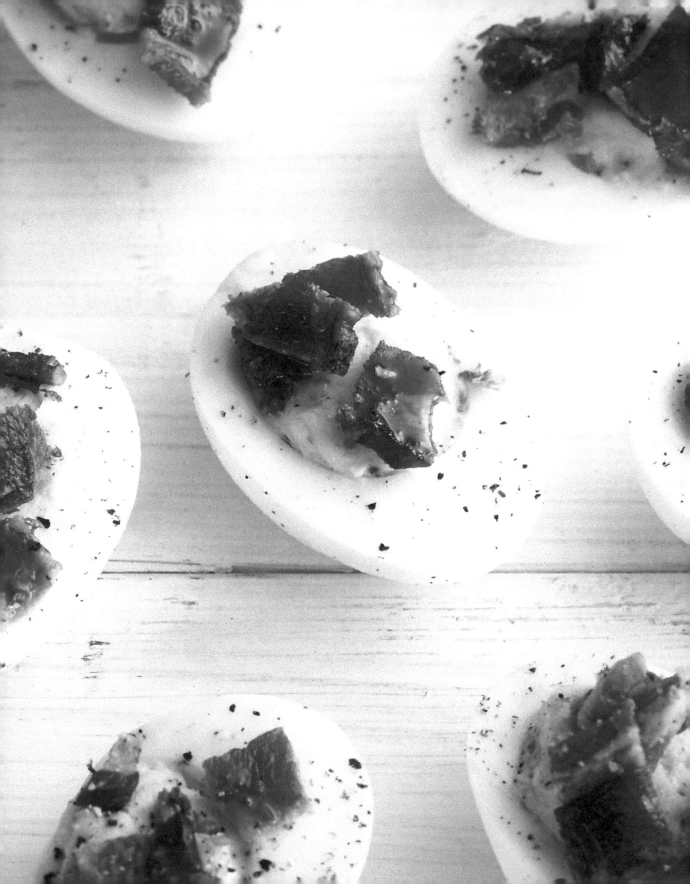

APPS & SNACKS

◀ Bacon-Cheese Deviled Eggs, page 66

BACON-PEPPER FAT BOMBS

Makes 12 fat bombs / Prep time: 10 minutes, plus 1 hour chilling time

Fat bombs are designed to help you reach your daily macros with no fuss and little planning required. This cheesy bacon bomb is savory and delectable, with a satisfying kick from the black pepper. If you want a little more heat, add a pinch of cayenne. It will definitely add a little pep to your step.

2 ounces goat cheese, at room temperature

2 ounces cream cheese, at room temperature

¼ cup butter, at room temperature

8 bacon slices, cooked and chopped

Pinch freshly ground black pepper

1. Line a small baking sheet with parchment paper and set aside.

2. In a medium bowl, stir together the goat cheese, cream cheese, butter, bacon, and pepper until well combined.

3. Use a tablespoon to drop mounds of the bomb mixture on the baking sheet and place the sheet in the freezer until the fat bombs are very firm but not frozen, about 1 hour.

4. Store the fat bombs in a sealed container in the refrigerator for up to 2 weeks.

PER SERVING (1 FAT BOMB) Calories: 89; Fat: 8g; Protein: 3g; Carbs: 0g; Fiber: 0g; Net Carbs: 0g; Fat 84%/Protein 15%/Carbs 1%

SMOKED SALMON FAT BOMBS

Makes 12 fat bombs / Prep time: 10 minutes, plus 2 hours chilling time

Many restaurants serve a popular appetizer that features smoked salmon and herb cream cheese spread on tortillas, rolled up, and cut into little bite size rounds. This keto version omits the tortillas but still has all the rich, delicious flavor. Add a sprinkle of chopped fresh dill into the mixture if it suits your taste.

½ cup goat cheese, at room temperature

½ cup butter, at room temperature

2 ounces smoked salmon

2 teaspoons freshly squeezed lemon juice

Pinch freshly ground black pepper

1. Line a baking sheet with parchment paper and set aside.

2. In a medium bowl, stir together the goat cheese, butter, smoked salmon, lemon juice, and pepper until very well blended.

3. Use a tablespoon to scoop the salmon mixture onto the baking sheet until you have 12 even mounds.

4. Place the baking sheet in the refrigerator until the fat bombs are firm, 2 to 3 hours.

5. Store the fat bombs in a sealed container in the refrigerator for up to 1 week.

A CLOSER LOOK Smoked salmon has more stable omega-3s than fresh fish, which means these healthy fats are less prone to oxidation. Look for better-quality smoked salmon because cheaper products are often smoked over sawdust.

PER SERVING (2 FAT BOMBS) Calories: 193; Fat: 18g; Protein: 8g; Carbs: 0g; Fiber: 0g; Net Carbs: 0g; Fat 84%/Protein 16%/Carbs 0%

WALNUT HERB-CRUSTED GOAT CHEESE

Serves 4 / Prep time: 10 minutes

Goat cheese is a marvelous tart creation that has about 12 grams of fat, 10 grams of protein, and zero carbs in a 2-ounce portion, which is the recommended serving size in this recipe. Try to find soft goat cheese because semihard and hard types actually do contain carbs. The soft product can be found in most grocery stores in prepackaged logs.

6 ounces chopped walnuts

1 tablespoon chopped oregano

1 tablespoon chopped parsley

1 teaspoon chopped fresh thyme

¼ teaspoon freshly ground black pepper

1 (8-ounce) log goat cheese

1. Place the walnuts, oregano, parsley, thyme, and pepper in a food processor and pulse until finely chopped.

2. Pour the walnut mixture onto a plate and roll the goat cheese log in the nut mixture, pressing so the cheese is covered and the walnut mixture sticks to the log.

3. Wrap the cheese in plastic and store in the refrigerator for up to 1 week.

4. Slice and enjoy!

PER SERVING Calories: 304; Fat: 28g; Protein: 12g; Carbs: 4g; Fiber: 2g; Net Carbs: 2g; Fat 77%/Protein 18%/ Carbs 6%

CRISPY PARMESAN CRACKERS

GLUTEN FREE
NUT FREE
VEGETARIAN
UNDER 30 MINUTES

Makes 8 crackers / Prep time: 10 minutes / Cook time: 5 minutes

Parmesan cheese has a nice keto ratio, especially when combined with a little butter to create these lacy beauties. The cheese spreads out and melts into large crispy golden crackers that will satisfy any craving for a rich savory treat. You can use grated Parmesan as well, as long as it is freshly grated. The pregrated cheese you'll find on supermarket shelves won't cut it—it tends to be too dry and powdery to melt correctly.

1 teaspoon butter

8 ounces full-fat Parmesan cheese, shredded or freshly grated

1. Preheat the oven to 400°F.
2. Line a baking sheet with parchment paper and lightly grease the paper with the butter.
3. Spoon the Parmesan cheese onto the baking sheet in mounds, spread evenly apart.
4. Spread out the mounds with the back of a spoon until they are flat.
5. Bake the crackers until the edges are browned and the centers are still pale, about 5 minutes.
6. Remove the sheet from the oven, and remove the crackers with a spatula to paper towels. Lightly blot the tops with additional paper towels and let them completely cool.
7. Store in a sealed container in the refrigerator for up to 4 days.

PER SERVING (1 CRACKER) Calories: 133; Fat: 11g; Protein: 11g; Carbs: 1g; Fiber: 0g; Net Carbs: 1g; Fat 70%/Protein 29%/Carbs 1%

BACON-CHEESE DEVILED EGGS

Makes 12 / Prep time: 15 minutes

A simple favorite is made extra special with the addition of bacon and tasty Swiss cheese. Eggs are a wonderful addition to the keto diet because they are an excellent source of fat and protein, about 63 percent and 35 percent, respectively, in one large egg. Deviled eggs can be eaten as a quick snack or taken to a get-together on a pretty platter for everyone to enjoy.

6 large eggs, hardboiled
  and peeled
¼ cup Creamy Mayonnaise
  (page 137)
¼ avocado, chopped

¼ cup Swiss cheese,
  finely shredded
½ teaspoon Dijon mustard
Freshly ground black pepper
6 bacon slices, cooked
  and chopped

1. Halve each of the eggs lengthwise.
2. Carefully remove the yolk and place the yolks in a medium bowl. Place the whites, hollow-side up, on a plate.
3. Mash the yolks with a fork and add the mayonnaise, avocado, cheese, and Dijon mustard. Stir until well mixed. Season the yolk mixture with the black pepper.
4. Spoon the yolk mixture back into the egg white hollows and top each egg half with the chopped bacon.
5. Store the eggs in an airtight container in the refrigerator for up to 1 day.

PREP TIP Hardboiled eggs make perfect snacks and a great addition to many recipes such as salads and entrees. Hardboil a dozen eggs at the beginning of the week and keep them in the refrigerator for when you need them.

PER SERVING (1 DEVILED EGG) Calories: 85; Fat: 7g; Protein: 6g; Carbs: 2g; Fiber: 0g; Net Carbs: 2g; Fat 70%/Protein 25%/Carbs 5%

QUESO DIP

Serves 6 / Prep time: 5 minutes / Cook time: 10 minutes

Also known as chile con queso, this dip originated in Mexico and can be found in many places that serve Tex-Mex cuisine. Jalapeño peppers are hot because they contain capsaicin. They are considered about medium in heat on the Scoville scale, with about 2,500 to 8,000 heat units per pepper. If you want a hotter dip, choose a pepper with more heat units, such as a habanero or Scotch bonnet chile.

½ cup coconut milk

½ jalapeño pepper, seeded and diced

1 teaspoon minced garlic

½ teaspoon onion powder

2 ounces goat cheese

6 ounces sharp Cheddar cheese, shredded

¼ teaspoon cayenne pepper

1. Place a medium pot over medium heat and add the coconut milk, jalapeño, garlic, and onion powder.

2. Bring the liquid to a simmer and then whisk in the goat cheese until smooth.

3. Add the Cheddar cheese and cayenne and whisk until the dip is thick, 30 seconds to 1 minute.

4. Pour into a serving dish and serve with keto crackers or low-carb vegetables.

PER SERVING Calories: 213; Fat: 19g; Protein: 10g; Carbs: 2g; Fiber: 0g; Net Carbs: 2g; Fat 79%/Protein 19%/Carbs 2%

CAULIFLOWER-CHEDDAR SOUP

Serves 8 / Prep time: 10 minutes / Cook time: 30 minutes

Cauliflower is a versatile vegetable that can be eaten on the keto diet in many recipes—like this creamy soup. Cauliflower is an excellent source of vitamins C and K, omega-3 fatty acids, and manganese, which can help support digestion, improve brain function, and promote a healthy heart. Choose a snowy white head of cauliflower with crisp green leaves and absolutely no brown spots.

¼ cup butter

½ sweet onion, chopped

1 head cauliflower, chopped

4 cups Herbed Chicken Stock (page 141)

½ teaspoon ground nutmeg

1 cup heavy (whipping) cream

Sea salt

Freshly ground black pepper

1 cup shredded Cheddar cheese

1. Put a large stockpot over medium heat and add the butter.

2. Sauté the onion and cauliflower until tender and lightly browned, about 10 minutes.

3. Add the chicken stock and nutmeg to the pot and bring the liquid to a boil.

4. Reduce the heat to low and simmer until the vegetables are very tender, about 15 minutes.

5. Remove the pot from the heat, stir in the heavy cream, and purée the soup with an immersion blender or food processor until smooth.

6. Season the soup with salt and pepper and serve topped with the Cheddar cheese.

PER SERVING Calories: 227; Fat: 21g; Protein: 8g; Carbs: 4g; Fiber: 2g; Net Carbs: 2g; Fat 81%/Protein 12%/Carbs 9%

BLT SALAD

Serves 4 / Prep time: 15 minutes

The portions of this salad are quite small, but the combination of ingredients packs a hearty flavor burst. Using bacon fat in the dressing instead of olive oil adds to this already mouthwatering salad. Bacon fat will keep in a sealed container in the refrigerator for up to 1 week, so save it for other recipes whenever you cook bacon.

2 tablespoons melted bacon fat

2 tablespoons red wine vinegar

Freshly ground black pepper

4 cups shredded lettuce

1 tomato, chopped

6 bacon slices, cooked
    and chopped

2 hardboiled eggs, chopped

1 tablespoon roasted unsalted
    sunflower seeds

1 teaspoon toasted sesame seeds

1 cooked chicken breast, sliced
    (optional)

1. In a medium bowl, whisk together the bacon fat and vinegar until emulsified. Season with black pepper.

2. Add the lettuce and tomato to the bowl and toss the vegetables with the dressing.

3. Divide the salad between 4 plates and top each with equal amounts of bacon, egg, sunflower seeds, sesame seeds, and chicken (if using). Serve.

SUBSTITUTION TIP If you want to try a warm bacon salad dressing, gently warm the bacon fat before whisking in the vinegar. Swap out regular lettuce for kale or spinach; the more robust greens will hold up better in the dressing.

PER SERVING Calories: 228; Fat: 18g; Protein: 1g; Carbs: 4g; Fiber: 2g;
Net Carbs: 2g; Fat 76%/Protein 17%/Carbs 7%

CHICKEN-AVOCADO LETTUCE WRAPS

Serves 4 / Prep time: 10 minutes

Lettuce wraps are a spectacular method of enjoying sandwiches and toppings without adding undesirable carbs. The best lettuce to use is Boston, large red or green oak leaf, or romaine lettuce with the rib cut out. Cutting out the ribs allows you to roll the lettuce leaf without it cracking or ripping.

½ avocado, peeled and pitted
⅓ cup Creamy Mayonnaise (page 137)
1 teaspoon freshly squeezed lemon juice
2 teaspoons chopped fresh thyme

1 (6-ounce) cooked chicken breast, chopped
Sea salt
Freshly ground black pepper
8 large lettuce leaves
¼ cup chopped walnuts

1. In a medium bowl, mash the avocado with the mayonnaise, lemon juice, and thyme until well combined.
2. Stir in the chopped chicken and season the filling with salt and pepper.
3. Spoon the chicken salad into the lettuce leaves and top with the walnuts.
4. Serve 2 lettuce wraps per person.

PER SERVING Calories: 264; Fat: 20g; Protein: 12g; Carbs: 9g; Fiber: 3g; Net Carbs: 6g; Fat 70%/Protein 16%/Carbs 14%

CRAB SALAD–STUFFED AVOCADO

Serves 2 / Prep time: 20 minutes

KETO QUOTIENT

GLUTEN FREE
NUT FREE
UNDER 30 MINUTES

Depending on the size of your avocados, this decadent dish could be a filling snack or a light lunch. It's perfectly acceptable to use frozen crab if fresh is not available, but take care to look for real crab meat rather than cheaper imitation products. If using frozen crab, thaw it completely and squeeze out any extra liquid so that your salad isn't soggy.

1 avocado, peeled, halved lengthwise, and pitted

½ teaspoon freshly squeezed lemon juice

4½ ounces Dungeness crabmeat

½ cup cream cheese

¼ cup chopped red bell pepper

¼ cup chopped, peeled English cucumber

½ scallion, chopped

1 teaspoon chopped cilantro

Pinch sea salt

Freshly ground black pepper

1. Brush the cut edges of the avocado with the lemon juice and set the halves aside on a plate.

2. In a medium bowl, stir together the crabmeat, cream cheese, red pepper, cucumber, scallion, cilantro, salt, and pepper until well mixed.

3. Divide the crab mixture between the avocado halves and store them, covered with plastic wrap, in the refrigerator until you want to serve them, up to 2 days.

A CLOSER LOOK Dungeness crab is in season from about December to April; this is the best time frame to purchase this sweet crustacean. The Seafood Watch rates Dungeness crab as sustainable seafood.

PER SERVING Calories: 389; Fat: 31g; Protein: 19g; Carbs: 10g; Fiber: 5g; Net Carbs: 5g; Fat 70%/Protein 20%/Carbs 10%

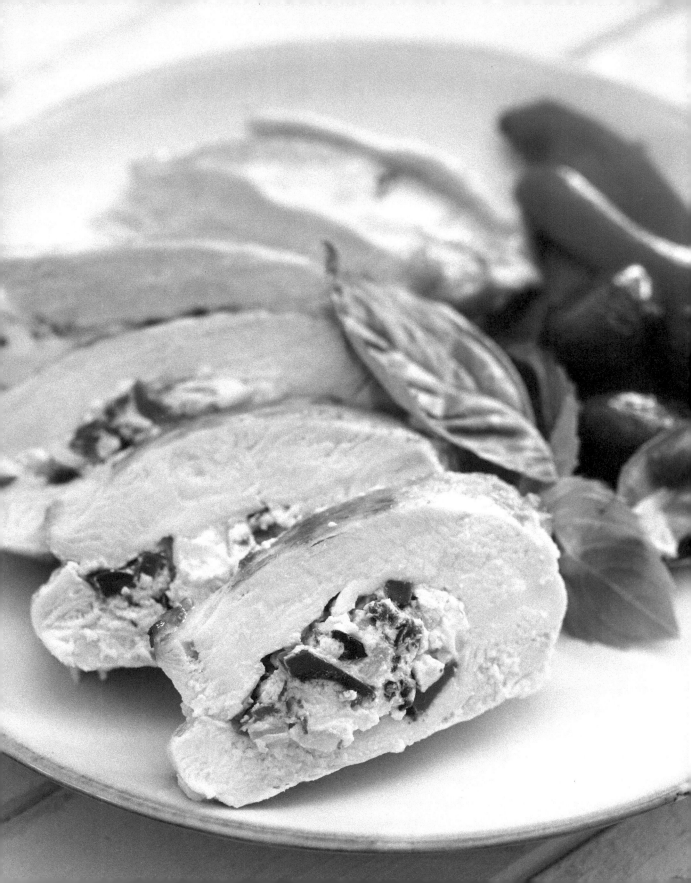

FISH & POULTRY

◀ Stuffed Chicken Breasts, page 86

SHRIMP AND SAUSAGE "BAKE"

Serves 4 / Prep time: 15 minutes / Cook time: 20 minutes

Chorizo, a fully cooked cured sausage common in Spanish, Portuguese, and Latin American cooking, can be either spicy or slightly sweet and has a distinctive red color from the copious amounts of paprika added during its creation. Chorizo is very high in protein, about 15 grams per 3-ounce portion, and is an excellent source of zinc, selenium, and vitamin B$_{12}$.

2 tablespoons olive oil

6 ounces chorizo sausage, diced

½ pound (16 to 20 count) shrimp, peeled and deveined

1 red bell pepper, chopped

½ small sweet onion, chopped

2 teaspoons minced garlic

¼ cup Herbed Chicken Stock (page 141)

Pinch red pepper flakes

1. Place a large skillet over medium-high heat and add the olive oil.
2. Sauté the sausage until it is warmed through, about 6 minutes.
3. Add the shrimp and sauté until it is opaque and just cooked through, about 4 minutes.
4. Remove the sausage and shrimp to a bowl and set aside.
5. Add the red pepper, onion, and garlic to the skillet and sauté until tender, about 4 minutes.
6. Add the chicken stock to the skillet along with the cooked sausage and shrimp.
7. Bring the liquid to a simmer and simmer for 3 minutes.
8. Stir in the red pepper flakes and serve.

A CLOSER LOOK Shrimp is often not sustainably caught, and most farmed shrimp are not considered to be very good for you. When purchasing shrimp, look for US wild-caught shrimp from the Pacific or southern areas or West Coast farmed shrimp from fully recirculating farms.

PER SERVING Calories: 323; Fat: 24g; Protein: 20g; Carbs: 8g; Fiber: 2g; Net Carbs: 6g; Fat 69%/Protein 25%/Carbs 6%

HERB BUTTER SCALLOPS

Serves 4 / Prep time: 10 minutes / Cook time: 10 minutes

KETO QUOTIENT

GLUTEN FREE
NUT FREE
UNDER 30 MINUTES

Scallops are usually placed squarely in the category of foods best enjoyed in a restaurant because this sweet seafood is thought to be difficult to cook. Scallops are actually quite easy to prepare if you watch them carefully and don't leave them on the heat too long. Scallops are very high in protein, selenium, and vitamin B_{12}. These nutrients are crucial for cardiovascular health and can help lower your risk of arthritis and colon cancer.

1 pound sea scallops, cleaned
Freshly ground black pepper
8 tablespoons butter, divided
2 teaspoons minced garlic

Juice of 1 lemon
2 teaspoons chopped fresh basil
1 teaspoon chopped fresh thyme

1. Pat the scallops dry with paper towels and season them lightly with pepper.
2. Place a large skillet over medium heat and add 2 tablespoons of butter.
3. Arrange the scallops in the skillet, evenly spaced but not too close together, and sear each side until they are golden brown, about 2½ minutes per side.
4. Remove the scallops to a plate and set aside.
5. Add the remaining 6 tablespoons of butter to the skillet and sauté the garlic until translucent, about 3 minutes.
6. Stir in the lemon juice, basil, and thyme and return the scallops to the skillet, turning to coat them in the sauce.
7. Serve immediately.

PER SERVING Calories: 306; Fat: 24g; Protein: 19g; Carbs: 4g; Fiber: 0g;
Net Carbs: 4g; Fat 70%/Protein 25%/Carbs 5%

PAN-SEARED HALIBUT WITH CITRUS BUTTER SAUCE

Serves 4 / Prep time: 10 minutes / Cook time: 15 minutes

Citrus fruits are absolutely delicious and are bursting with nutrients. Both lemons and oranges are excellent sources of vitamin C, which boosts the immune system and can help detoxify your body. The acid from citrus is a wonderful addition to most fish and seafood recipes.

4 (5-ounce) halibut fillets, each about 1 inch thick
Sea salt
Freshly ground black pepper
¼ cup butter
2 teaspoons minced garlic
1 shallot, minced

3 tablespoons dry white wine
1 tablespoon freshly squeezed lemon juice
1 tablespoon freshly squeezed orange juice
2 teaspoons chopped fresh parsley
2 tablespoons olive oil

1. Pat the fish dry with paper towels and then lightly season the fillets with salt and pepper. Set aside on a paper towel–lined plate.
2. Place a small saucepan over medium heat and melt the butter.
3. Sauté the garlic and shallot until tender, about 3 minutes.
4. Whisk in the white wine, lemon juice, and orange juice and bring the sauce to a simmer, cooking until it thickens slightly, about 2 minutes.
5. Remove the sauce from the heat and stir in the parsley; set aside.
6. Place a large skillet over medium-high heat and add the olive oil.
7. Panfry the fish until lightly browned and just cooked through, turning them over once, about 10 minutes in total.
8. Serve the fish immediately with a spoonful of sauce for each.

SUBSTITUTION TIP Any firm white-fleshed fish will be delicious with this creamy sauce. Try haddock, tilapia, or sea bass.

PER SERVING Calories: 319; Fat: 26g; Protein: 22g; Carbs: 2g; Fiber: 0g; Net Carbs: 2g; Fat 70%/Protein 29%/Carbs 1%

SIMPLE FISH CURRY

Serves 4 / Prep time: 10 minutes / Cook time: 25 minutes

Curry is a sauce-based recipe originating in India and adapted by many cultures. The ubiquitous spice mixture often contains a multitude of ingredients, such as cumin, coriander, turmeric, ginger, cloves, paprika, and cinnamon. It's adapted so well to many cuisines because no matter the ingredients used—vegetables, meats, fish, eggs, butter, coconut—the spices bring the dish together beautifully.

2 tablespoons coconut oil

1½ tablespoons grated
   fresh ginger

2 teaspoons minced garlic

1 tablespoon curry powder

½ teaspoon ground cumin

2 cups coconut milk

16 ounces firm white fish,
   cut into 1-inch chunks

1 cup shredded kale

2 tablespoons chopped cilantro

1. Place a large saucepan over medium heat and melt the coconut oil.

2. Sauté the ginger and garlic until lightly browned, about 2 minutes.

3. Stir in the curry powder and cumin and sauté until very fragrant, about 2 minutes.

4. Stir in the coconut milk and bring the liquid to a boil.

5. Reduce the heat to low and simmer for about 5 minutes to infuse the milk with the spices.

6. Add the fish and cook until the fish is cooked through, about 10 minutes.

7. Stir in the kale and cilantro and simmer until wilted, about 2 minutes.

8. Serve.

PER SERVING Calories: 416; Fat: 31g; Protein: 26g; Carbs: 5g; Fiber: 1g;
Net Carbs: 4g; Fat 70%/Protein 24%/Carbs 6%

ROASTED SALMON WITH AVOCADO SALSA

Serves 4 / Prep time: 15 minutes / Cook time: 12 minutes

A simple fresh salsa is often the best topping for a juicy piece of fish, and creamy avocados are a perfect choice for the base. Take the salsa ingredients out of the refrigerator an hour or so before serving the fish so they come to room temperature. The taste of the avocado will be much stronger than when this fruit is completely chilled. You can also grill the salmon for this recipe—this fish holds up well under higher heat and does not dry out.

FOR THE SALSA
1 avocado, peeled, pitted, and diced
1 scallion, white and green parts, chopped
½ cup halved cherry tomatoes
Juice of 1 lemon
Zest of 1 lemon

FOR THE FISH
1 teaspoon ground cumin
½ teaspoon ground coriander
½ teaspoon onion powder
¼ teaspoon sea salt
Pinch freshly ground black pepper
Pinch cayenne pepper
4 (4-ounce) boneless, skinless salmon fillets
2 tablespoons olive oil

TO MAKE THE SALSA

1. In a small bowl, stir together the avocado, scallion, tomatoes, lemon juice, and lemon zest until mixed.

2. Set aside.

TO MAKE THE FISH

1. Preheat the oven to 400°F. Line a baking sheet with aluminum foil and set aside.

2. In a small bowl, stir together the cumin, coriander, onion powder, salt, black pepper, and cayenne until well mixed.

3. Rub the salmon fillets with the spice mix and place them on the baking sheet.

4. Drizzle the fillets with the olive oil and roast the fish until it is just cooked through, about 15 minutes.

5. Serve the salmon topped with the avocado salsa.

PER SERVING Calories: 320; Fat: 26g; Protein: 22g; Carbs: 4g; Fiber: 3g; Net Carbs: 1g; Fat 69%/Protein 26%/Carbs 5%

SOLE ASIAGO

Serves 4 / Prep time: 10 minutes / Cook time: 8 minutes

Sole is a flat fish, which means both of its eyes are on one side of its head. It looks rather strange, but when filleted, it is delicious. Sole is not a threatened species, but it is overfished in some areas, so it is not as plentiful as it was in the past. This tender, delicate fish freezes very well; if you cannot find fresh fillets, frozen fillets will work, too.

4 (4-ounce) sole fillets

¾ cup ground almonds

¼ cup Asiago cheese

2 eggs, beaten

2½ tablespoons melted coconut oil

1. Preheat the oven to 350°F. Line a baking sheet with parchment paper and set aside.
2. Pat the fish dry with paper towels.
3. Stir together the ground almonds and cheese in a small bowl.
4. Place the bowl with the beaten eggs in it next to the almond mixture.
5. Dredge a sole fillet in the beaten egg and then press the fish into the almond mixture so it is completely coated. Place on the baking sheet and repeat until all the fillets are breaded.
6. Brush both sides of each piece of fish with the coconut oil.
7. Bake the sole until it is cooked through, about 8 minutes in total.
8. Serve immediately.

PER SERVING Calories: 406; Fat: 31g; Protein: 29g; Carbs: 6g; Fiber: 3g; Net Carbs: 3g; Fat 65%/Protein 30%/Carbs 5%

BAKED COCONUT HADDOCK

Serves 4 / Prep time: 10 minutes / Cook time: 12 minutes

KETO QUOTIENT

DAIRY FREE
GLUTEN FREE
UNDER 30 MINUTES

A lovely golden nut crust not only adds fabulous flavor to fish, it also helps prevent overcooking of the fillets so they stay moist. This protective coating can be any type of nut from delicate almonds to more robust pistachios. Just substitute the other nuts in the same amount as the hazelnuts in the recipe.

4 (5-ounce) boneless
   haddock fillets
Sea salt
Freshly ground black pepper

1 cup shredded unsweetened
   coconut
¼ cup ground hazelnuts
2 tablespoons coconut oil, melted

1. Preheat the oven to 400°F. Line a baking sheet with parchment paper and set aside.

2. Pat the fillets very dry with paper towels and lightly season them with salt and pepper.

3. Stir together the shredded coconut and hazelnuts in a small bowl.

4. Dredge the fish fillets in the coconut mixture so that both sides of each piece are thickly coated.

5. Place the fish on the baking sheet and lightly brush both sides of each piece with the coconut oil.

6. Bake the haddock until the topping is golden and the fish flakes easily with a fork, about 12 minutes total.

7. Serve.

PREP TIP The breading of the fish can be done ahead, up to 1 day, if you just want to pop the fish in the oven when you get home. Place the breaded fish on the baking sheet and cover it with plastic wrap in the refrigerator until you wish to bake it.

PER SERVING Calories: 299; Fat: 24g; Protein: 20g; Carbs: 4g; Fiber: 3g; Net Carbs: 1g; Fat 66%/Protein 28%/Carbs 6%

CHEESY GARLIC SALMON

Serves 4 / Prep time: 15 minutes / Cook time: 12 minutes

Salmon has such a satisfying firm texture and strong flavor that it can handle the garlic and cheese in this dish. Salmon is one of the healthiest fish choices, with loads of nutrients such as vitamin D and omega-3 fatty acids. Wild salmon caught in the Pacific off the US and Canadian coasts have a very high level of these disease-busting anti-inflammatory nutrients and antioxidants.

½ cup Asiago cheese

2 tablespoons freshly squeezed lemon juice

2 tablespoons butter, at room temperature

2 teaspoons minced garlic

1 teaspoon chopped fresh basil

1 teaspoon chopped fresh oregano

4 (5-ounce) salmon fillets

1 tablespoon olive oil

1. Preheat the oven to 350°F. Line a baking sheet with parchment paper and set aside.

2. In a small bowl, stir together the Asiago cheese, lemon juice, butter, garlic, basil, and oregano.

3. Pat the salmon dry with paper towels and place the fillets on the baking sheet skin-side down. Divide the topping evenly between the fillets and spread it across the fish using a knife or the back of a spoon.

4. Drizzle the fish with the olive oil and bake until the topping is golden and the fish is just cooked through, about 12 minutes.

5. Serve.

PER SERVING Calories: 357; Fat: 28g; Protein: 24g; Carbs: 2g; Fiber: 0g; Net Carbs: 2g; Fat 70%/Protein 28%/Carbs 2%

LEMON BUTTER CHICKEN

Serves 4 / Prep time: 10 minutes / Cook time: 40 minutes

Chicken is a staple food in many households because it combines so well with many other ingredients and its mild flavor is a favorite even among picky eaters. If your budget allows, look for organic grass-fed chicken at your local grocery store because it tastes better than the meat from factory-farmed birds. Organic grass-fed chicken also contains more vitamin A and omega-3 fatty acids.

4 bone-in, skin-on chicken thighs
Sea salt
Freshly ground black pepper
2 tablespoons butter, divided
2 teaspoons minced garlic

½ cup Herbed Chicken Stock
(page 141)
½ cup heavy (whipping) cream
Juice of ½ lemon

1. Preheat the oven to 400°F.
2. Lightly season the chicken thighs with salt and pepper.
3. Place a large ovenproof skillet over medium-high heat and add 1 tablespoon of butter.
4. Brown the chicken thighs until golden on both sides, about 6 minutes in total. Remove the thighs to a plate and set aside.
5. Add the remaining 1 tablespoon of butter and sauté the garlic until translucent, about 2 minutes.
6. Whisk in the chicken stock, heavy cream, and lemon juice.
7. Bring the sauce to a boil and then return the chicken to the skillet.
8. Place the skillet in the oven, covered, and braise until the chicken is cooked through, about 30 minutes.

A CLOSER LOOK Chicken thighs often get overlooked when next to the more popular breasts, but they have more flavor and are juicier. Thighs are also less expensive than chicken breasts and are a smart choice at least once per week for people on a budget.

PER SERVING Calories: 294; Fat: 26g; Protein: 12g; Carbs: 4g; Fiber: 1g;
Net Carbs: 3g; Fat 78%/Protein 17%/Carbs 5%

CHICKEN BACON BURGERS

Serves 6 / Prep time: 10 minutes / Cook time: 25 minutes

The absolute best method of cooking these juicy herbed burgers is over a medium-heat grill, but this oven-baked recipe works very well too. You might want to double the batch and place the formed burgers in the freezer between parchment paper layers and tightly wrapped in plastic, or placed in a sealed freezer bag. Simply thaw and cook for an easy dinner at a later time.

1 pound ground chicken

8 bacon slices, chopped

¼ cup ground almonds

1 teaspoon chopped fresh basil

¼ teaspoon sea salt

Pinch freshly ground black pepper

2 tablespoons coconut oil

4 large lettuce leaves

1 avocado, peeled, pitted, and sliced

1. Preheat the oven to 350°F. Line a baking sheet with parchment paper and set aside.

2. In a medium bowl, combine the chicken, bacon, ground almonds, basil, salt, and pepper until well mixed.

3. Form the mixture into 6 equal patties.

4. Place a large skillet over medium-high heat and add the coconut oil.

5. Pan sear the chicken patties until brown on both sides, about 6 minutes in total.

6. Place the browned patties on the baking sheet and bake until completely cooked through, about 15 minutes.

7. Serve on the lettuce leaves, topped with the avocado slices.

PER SERVING Calories: 374; Fat: 33g; Protein: 18g; Carbs: 3g; Fiber: 2g; Net Carbs: 1g; Fat 78%/Protein 20%/Carbs 2%

PAPRIKA CHICKEN

Serves 4 / Prep time: 10 minutes / Cook time: 25 minutes

KETO QUOTIENT

GLUTEN FREE
NUT FREE

Paprika is a glorious red spice created by grinding dried sweet red bell peppers and chile peppers into a fine powder. It's available in sweet, hot, and smoked varieties, to name just a few. The rich color and piquant flavor of paprika infuses the other ingredients in this recipe. Paprika also adds some health benefits to the recipe, such as protecting the eyes from macular degeneration.

4 (4-ounce) chicken breasts, skin-on
Sea salt
Freshly ground black pepper
1 tablespoon olive oil
½ cup chopped sweet onion

½ cup heavy (whipping) cream
2 teaspoons smoked paprika
½ cup sour cream
2 tablespoons chopped fresh parsley

1. Lightly season the chicken with salt and pepper.
2. Place a large skillet over medium-high heat and add the olive oil.
3. Sear the chicken on both sides until almost cooked through, about 15 minutes in total. Remove the chicken to a plate.
4. Add the onion to the skillet and sauté until tender, about 4 minutes.
5. Stir in the cream and paprika and bring the liquid to a simmer.
6. Return the chicken and any accumulated juices to the skillet and simmer the chicken for 5 minutes until completely cooked.
7. Stir in the sour cream and remove the skillet from the heat.
8. Serve topped with the parsley.

PER SERVING Calories: 389; Fat: 30g; Protein: 25g; Carbs: 4g; Fiber: 0g; Net Carbs: 4g; Fat 70%/Protein 26%/Carbs 4%

STUFFED CHICKEN BREASTS

Serves 4 / Prep time: 30 minutes, plus 30 minutes chilling time /
Cook time: 30 minutes

This dish might perfectly complement a complicated risotto in a fancy fine-dining restaurant. The trick to perfect stuffed chicken breasts is to cut a perfect pocket— not too deep but with enough space so the filling is completely enclosed. If it isn't enclosed, the filling will simply melt in the oven, leaving an empty pocket.

1 tablespoon butter

¼ cup chopped sweet onion

½ cup goat cheese, at room temperature

¼ cup Kalamata olives, chopped

¼ cup chopped roasted red pepper

2 tablespoons chopped fresh basil

4 (5-ounce) chicken breasts, skin-on

2 tablespoons extra-virgin olive oil

1. Preheat the oven to 400°F.

2. In a small skillet over medium heat, melt the butter and add the onion. Sauté until tender, about 3 minutes.

3. Transfer the onion to a medium bowl and add the cheese, olives, red pepper, and basil. Stir until well blended, then refrigerate for about 30 minutes.

4. Cut horizontal pockets into each chicken breast, and stuff them evenly with the filling. Secure the two sides of each breast with toothpicks.

5. Place a large ovenproof skillet over medium-high heat and add the olive oil.

6. Brown the chicken on both sides, about 10 minutes in total.

7. Place the skillet in the oven and roast until the chicken is just cooked through, about 15 minutes. Remove the toothpicks and serve.

SUBSTITUTION TIP If fresh basil is not available in the grocery store or your garden, try using a premade paste or frozen basil in the filling. You can also use a spoon of pesto for added flavor.

PER SERVING Calories: 389; Fat: 30g; Protein: 25g; Carbs: 3g; Fiber: 0g; Net Carbs: 3g; Fat 70%/Protein 28%/Carbs 2%

COCONUT CHICKEN

Serves 4 / Prep time: 15 minutes / Cook time: 25 minutes

One of the main components of this recipe is rich, creamy coconut milk, which is a popular keto ingredient. The various types of coconut milk available might be confusing, but the best is the canned variety with a thick layer of coconut cream on top. Either stir the cream into the milk or skim it off for other recipes after opening the can.

2 tablespoons olive oil

4 (4-ounce) chicken breasts, cut into 2-inch chunks

½ cup chopped sweet onion

1 cup coconut milk

1 tablespoon curry powder

1 teaspoon ground cumin

1 teaspoon ground coriander

¼ cup chopped fresh cilantro

1. Place a large saucepan over medium-high heat and add the olive oil.

2. Sauté the chicken until almost cooked through, about 10 minutes.

3. Add the onion and sauté for an additional 3 minutes.

4. In a medium bowl, whisk together the coconut milk, curry powder, cumin, and coriander.

5. Pour the sauce into the saucepan with the chicken and bring the liquid to a boil.

6. Reduce the heat and simmer until the chicken is tender and the sauce has thickened, about 10 minutes.

7. Serve the chicken with the sauce, topped with cilantro.

PER SERVING Calories: 382; Fat: 31g; Protein: 23g; Carbs: 5g; Fiber: 1g; Net Carbs: 4g; Fat 70%/Protein 26%/Carbs 4%

TURKEY MEATLOAF

Serves 6 / Prep time: 10 minutes / Cook time: 35 minutes

Good meatloaf is an art and a successful staple dish for many home cooks. It is one of the ultimate comfort foods. Meatloaf needs the perfect ratio of meat, fats, vegetables, and spices to be tender and flavorful. The best part about meatloaf is that it freezes beautifully, so you can make a double batch and keep one for a quick meal at another time.

1 tablespoon olive oil
½ sweet onion, chopped
1½ pounds ground turkey
⅓ cup heavy (whipping) cream
¼ cup freshly grated Parmesan cheese

1 tablespoon chopped fresh parsley
Pinch sea salt
Pinch freshly ground black pepper

1. Heat the oven to 450°F.
2. Place a small skillet over medium heat and add the olive oil.
3. Sauté the onion until it is tender, about 4 minutes.
4. Transfer the onion to a large bowl and add the turkey, heavy cream, Parmesan cheese, parsley, salt, and pepper.
5. Stir until the ingredients are combined and hold together. Press the mixture into a loaf pan.
6. Bake until cooked through, about 30 minutes.
7. Let the meatloaf rest for 10 minutes and serve.

PER SERVING Calories: 216; Fat: 19g; Protein: 15g; Carbs: 1g; Fiber: 0g; Net Carbs: 1g; Fat 69%/Protein 29%/Carbs 2%

TURKEY RISSOLES

Serves 4 / Prep time: 10 minutes / Cook time: 25 minutes

Chicken is often the first choice for poultry in most home kitchens, but turkey is fabulous tasting, inexpensive, and very healthy. Turkey is low in fat and high in protein. Make sure some of your other recipe ingredients are high in fat so your keto macro is perfect. Turkey can help boost your immunity because it contains an amino acid called tryptophan, which supports the immune system.

1 pound ground turkey

1 scallion, white and green parts, finely chopped

1 teaspoon minced garlic

Pinch sea salt

Pinch freshly ground black pepper

1 cup ground almonds

2 tablespoons olive oil

1. Preheat the oven to 350°F. Line a baking sheet with aluminum foil and set aside.

2. In a medium bowl, mix together the turkey, scallion, garlic, salt, and pepper until well combined.

3. Shape the turkey mixture into 8 patties and flatten them out.

4. Place the ground almonds in a shallow bowl and dredge the turkey patties in the ground almonds to coat.

5. Place a large skillet over medium heat and add the olive oil.

6. Brown the turkey patties on both sides, about 10 minutes in total.

7. Transfer the patties to the baking sheet and bake them until cooked through, flipping them once, about 15 minutes in total.

PREP TIP Make the entire recipe from start to finish and place the cooled turkey patties in sealed plastic bags and store them in the refrigerator for up to 3 days or the freezer for up to 1 month. Take them out of the freezer and thaw for a quick dinner or snack or reheat them right from the refrigerator.

PER SERVING Calories: 440; Fat: 34g; Protein: 27g; Carbs: 7g; Fiber: 4g; Net Carbs: 3g; Fat 70%/Protein 25%/Carbs 5%

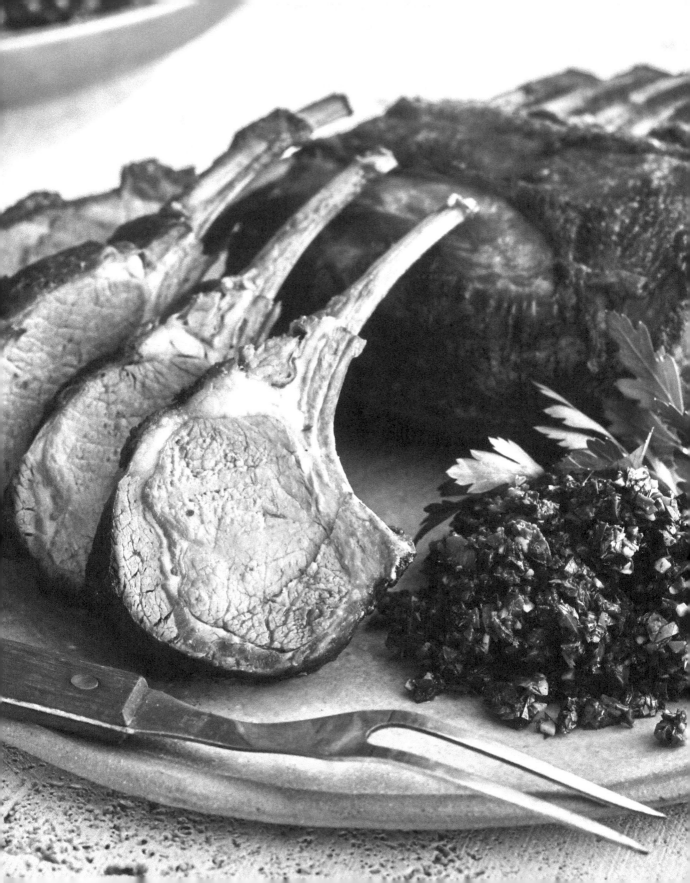

MEATS

◀ Lamb Chops with Kalamata Tapenade, page 94

NUT-STUFFED PORK CHOPS

Serves 4 / Prep time: 20 minutes / Cook time: 30 minutes

Pork is a healthy choice that falls somewhere between poultry and red meat on the nutrition spectrum, which is why pork is often called the other white meat. Pork is very high in protein and vitamin D and low in saturated fat. You will have to combine pork with ingredients higher in fat, like the nuts and goat cheese in this recipe, to meet your keto macros.

3 ounces goat cheese
½ cup chopped walnuts
¼ cup toasted chopped almonds
1 teaspoon chopped fresh thyme

4 center-cut pork chops, butterflied
Sea salt
Freshly ground black pepper
2 tablespoons olive oil

1. Preheat the oven to 400°F.
2. In a small bowl, make the filling by stirring together the goat cheese, walnuts, almonds, and thyme until well mixed.
3. Season the pork chops inside and outside with salt and pepper. Stuff each chop, pushing the filling to the bottom of the cut section. Secure the stuffing with toothpicks through the meat.
4. Place a large skillet over medium-high heat and add the olive oil. Pan sear the pork chops until they're browned on each side, about 10 minutes in total.
5. Transfer the pork chops to a baking dish and roast the chops in the oven until cooked through, about 20 minutes.
6. Serve after removing the toothpicks.

PER SERVING Calories: 481; Fat: 38g; Protein: 29g; Carbs: 5g; Fiber: 3g; Net Carbs: 2g; Fat 70%/Protein 25%/Carbs 5%

ROASTED PORK LOIN WITH GRAINY MUSTARD SAUCE

Serves 8 / Prep time: 10 minutes / Cook time: 70 minutes

This sauce is delicious; you might have to double the amount you make because eating it by the spoonful as a snack is a real treat. It is also stellar with barbecued beef tenderloin or a perfectly roasted lamb rack.

1 (2-pound) boneless pork
  loin roast
Sea salt
Freshly ground black pepper

3 tablespoons olive oil
1½ cups heavy (whipping) cream
3 tablespoons grainy mustard,
  such as Pommery

1. Preheat the oven to 375°F.
2. Season the pork roast all over with sea salt and pepper.
3. Place a large skillet over medium-high heat and add the olive oil.
4. Brown the roast on all sides in the skillet, about 6 minutes in total, and place the roast in a baking dish.
5. Roast until a meat thermometer inserted in the thickest part of the roast reads 155°F, about 1 hour.
6. When there is approximately 15 minutes of roasting time left, place a small saucepan over medium heat and add the heavy cream and mustard.
7. Stir the sauce until it simmers, then reduce the heat to low. Simmer the sauce until it is very rich and thick, about 5 minutes. Remove the pan from the heat and set aside.
8. Let the pork rest for 10 minutes before slicing and serve with the sauce.

A CLOSER LOOK Look for Pommery mustard, which is slightly sweet and adds a lovely burst of flavor to this decadent sauce.

PER SERVING Calories: 368; Fat: 29g; Protein: 25g; Carbs: 2g; Fiber: 0g; Net Carbs: 2g; Fat 70%/Protein 25%/Carbs 5%

KETO QUOTIENT

DAIRY FREE
GLUTEN FREE
NUT FREE

LAMB CHOPS WITH KALAMATA TAPENADE

Serves 4 / Prep time: 15 minutes / Cook time: 25 minutes

Lamb racks seem like the epitome of fine dining, perfectly cooked and cut into chops that are arranged in patterns with elegant bones pointing to the ceiling. Frenching the racks—removing the meat from the upper bones cleanly—is not difficult but can certainly be time consuming if you have never done it before. If you get the racks from your local butcher, you can always ask them to do the work for you to save valuable kitchen time.

FOR THE TAPENADE
1 cup pitted Kalamata olives
2 tablespoons chopped
   fresh parsley
2 tablespoons extra-virgin
   olive oil
2 teaspoons minced garlic
2 teaspoons freshly squeezed
   lemon juice

FOR THE LAMB CHOPS
2 (1-pound) racks French-cut
   lamb chops (8 bones each)
Sea salt
Freshly ground black pepper
1 tablespoon olive oil

TO MAKE THE TAPENADE

1. Place the olives, parsley, olive oil, garlic, and lemon juice in a food processor and process until the mixture is puréed but still slightly chunky.

2. Transfer the tapenade to a container and store sealed in the refrigerator until needed.

TO MAKE THE LAMB CHOPS

1. Preheat the oven to 450°F.

2. Season the lamb racks with salt and pepper.

3. Place a large ovenproof skillet over medium-high heat and add the olive oil.

4. Pan sear the lamb racks on all sides until browned, about 5 minutes in total.

5. Arrange the racks upright in the skillet, with the bones interlaced, and roast them in the oven until they reach your desired doneness, about 20 minutes for medium-rare or until the internal temperature reaches 125°F.

6. Let the lamb rest for 10 minutes and then cut the lamb racks into chops. Arrange 4 chops per person on the plate and top with the Kalamata tapenade.

SUBSTITUTION TIP Kalamata olives are grown in Greece and are a glorious purple-black color. Keep an eye out for unusual olives to try with this recipe, and try to avoid the standard canned black olives, which are often processed unripe fruit.

PER SERVING Calories: 348; Fat: 28g; Protein: 21g; Carbs: 2g; Fiber: 1g; Net Carbs: 1g; Fat 72%/Protein 25%/Carbs 3%

ROSEMARY-GARLIC LAMB RACKS

Serves 4 / Prep time: 10 minutes, plus 1 hour marinating time / Cook time: 25 minutes

Lamb is not one of the most popular meat choices in North America, but it is consumed in many other countries as a staple food. Spring lamb is the best choice when considering this product, although you can find lamb both fresh and frozen year-round in most grocery stores. If you are using frozen lamb, make sure it is completely thawed before adding the racks to the marinade.

4 tablespoons extra-virgin olive oil

2 tablespoons finely chopped
  fresh rosemary

2 teaspoons minced garlic

Pinch sea salt

2 (1-pound) racks French-cut
  lamb chops (8 bones each)

1. In a small bowl, whisk together the olive oil, rosemary, garlic, and salt.
2. Place the racks in a sealable freezer bag and pour the olive oil mixture into the bag. Massage the meat through the bag so it is coated with the marinade. Press the air out of the bag and seal it.
3. Marinate the lamb racks in the refrigerator for 1 to 2 hours.
4. Preheat the oven to 450°F.
5. Place a large ovenproof skillet over medium-high heat. Take the lamb racks out of the bag and sear them in the skillet on all sides, about 5 minutes in total.
6. Arrange the racks upright in the skillet, with the bones interlaced, and roast them in the oven until they reach your desired doneness, about 20 minutes for medium-rare or until the internal temperature reaches 125°F.
7. Let the lamb rest for 10 minutes and then cut the racks into chops.
8. Serve 4 chops per person.

PER SERVING Calories: 354; Fat: 30g; Protein: 21g; Carbs: 0g; Fiber: 0g; Net Carbs: 0g; Fat 70%/Protein 30%/Carbs 0%

LAMB LEG WITH SUN-DRIED TOMATO PESTO

Serves 8 / Prep time: 15 minutes / Cook time: 70 minutes

Sun-dried tomatoes, especially those packed in seasoned olive oil, provide an intense burst of flavor and are perfect for pesto and sauces. The drying process removes the tomatoes' water content while retaining and amplifying most of the nutrients and sweet taste of this popular fruit. Sun-dried tomatoes are an excellent source of iron, vitamin K, and protein.

FOR THE PESTO

1 cup sun-dried tomatoes packed
   in oil, drained
¼ cup pine nuts
2 tablespoons extra-virgin olive oil
2 tablespoons chopped fresh basil
2 teaspoons minced garlic

FOR THE LAMB LEG

1 (2-pound) lamb leg
Sea salt
Freshly ground black pepper
2 tablespoons olive oil

TO MAKE THE PESTO

1. Place the sun-dried tomatoes, pine nuts, olive oil, basil, and garlic in a blender or food processor, process until smooth.

2. Set aside until needed.

TO MAKE THE LAMB LEG

1. Preheat the oven to 400°F.

2. Season the lamb leg all over with salt and pepper.

3. Place a large ovenproof skillet over medium-high heat and add the olive oil.

4. Sear the lamb on all sides until nicely browned, about 6 minutes in total.

5. Spread the sun-dried tomato pesto all over the lamb and place the lamb on a baking sheet. Roast until the meat reaches your desired doneness, about 1 hour for medium.

6. Let the lamb rest for 10 minutes before slicing and serving.

PER SERVING Calories: 352; Fat: 29g; Protein: 17g; Carbs: 5g; Fiber: 2g; Net Carbs: 3g; Fat 74%/Protein 20%/Carbs 6%

SIRLOIN WITH BLUE CHEESE COMPOUND BUTTER

Serves 4 / Prep time: 10 minutes, plus 1 hour chilling time / Cook time: 12 minutes

Compound butters—butter mixed with another ingredient such as an herb or a cheese—are an easy, quick way to get intense flavor in your recipes. The heat of the prepared meats, poultry, or vegetables melts the butter into a scrumptious pool with no work beyond cutting a disk of butter off the prepared log. Compound butters will keep in the freezer, tightly wrapped, for up to a month.

6 tablespoons butter, at room temperature

4 ounces blue cheese, such as Stilton or Roquefort

4 (5-ounce) beef sirloin steaks

1 tablespoon olive oil

Sea salt

Freshly ground black pepper

1. Place the butter in a blender and pulse until the butter is whipped, about 2 minutes.

2. Add the cheese and pulse until just incorporated.

3. Spoon the butter mixture onto a sheet of plastic wrap and roll it into a log about 1½ inches in diameter by twisting both ends of the plastic wrap in opposite directions.

4. Refrigerate the butter until completely set, about 1 hour.

5. Slice the butter into ½-inch disks and set them on a plate in the refrigerator until you are ready to serve the steaks. Store leftover butter in the refrigerator for up to 1 week.

6. Preheat a barbecue to medium-high heat.

7. Let the steaks come to room temperature.

8. Rub the steaks all over with the olive oil and season them with salt and pepper.

9. Grill the steaks until they reach your desired doneness, about 6 minutes per side for medium.

10. If you do not have a barbecue, broil the steaks in a preheated oven for 7 minutes per side for medium.

11. Let the steaks rest for 10 minutes. Serve each topped with a disk of the compound butter.

PER SERVING Calories: 544; Fat: 44g; Protein: 35g; Carbs: 0g; Fiber: 0g; Net Carbs: 0g; Fat 72%/Protein 28%/Carbs 0%

GARLIC-BRAISED SHORT RIBS

KETO QUOTIENT

DAIRY FREE
GLUTEN FREE
NUT FREE

Serves 4 / Prep time: 10 minutes / Cook time: 2 hours, 20 minutes

Garlic infuses these ribs with a complex flavor and adds a plethora of important nutrients, because this allium is the source of about 70 phytochemicals, calcium, selenium, and manganese. Garlic has been used for centuries as a medicinal ingredient for its detoxing qualities and to lower blood pressure. Including garlic as a regular part of your diet is even thought to cut your risk of getting the common cold.

4 (4-ounce) beef short ribs
Sea salt
Freshly ground black pepper
1 tablespoon olive oil

2 teaspoons minced garlic
½ cup dry red wine
3 cups Rich Beef Stock (page 138)

1. Preheat the oven to 325°F.
2. Season the beef ribs on all sides with salt and pepper.
3. Place a deep ovenproof skillet over medium-high heat and add the olive oil.
4. Sear the ribs on all sides until browned, about 6 minutes in total. Transfer the ribs to a plate.
5. Add the garlic to the skillet and sauté until translucent, about 3 minutes.
6. Whisk in the red wine to deglaze the pan. Be sure to scrape all the browned bits from the meat from the bottom of the pan. Simmer the wine until it is slightly reduced, about 2 minutes.
7. Add the beef stock, ribs, and any accumulated juices on the plate back to the skillet and bring the liquid to a boil.
8. Cover the skillet and place it in the oven to braise the ribs until the meat is fall-off-the-bone tender, about 2 hours.
9. Serve the ribs with a spoonful of the cooking liquid drizzled over each serving.

PER SERVING Calories: 481; Fat: 38g; Protein: 29g; Carbs: 5g; Fiber: 3g; Net Carbs: 2g; Fat 70%/Protein 25%/Carbs 5%

BACON-WRAPPED BEEF TENDERLOIN

KETO QUOTIENT

DAIRY FREE
GLUTEN FREE
NUT FREE
UNDER 30 MINUTES

Serves 4 / Prep time: 10 minutes / Cook time: 15 minutes

This is a throwback to a popular '80s dish, when many things were wrapped in bacon despite the moratorium on fats. Bacon-wrapped steaks were found on every restaurant menu because the salty richness of the bacon combined beautifully with the lean tenderloin. If you are looking for higher omega-3 fatty acids and vitamin E in your beef, source-out organic grass-fed animals.

4 (4-ounce) beef tenderloin steaks

Sea salt

Freshly ground black pepper

8 bacon slices

1 tablespoon extra-virgin olive oil

1. Preheat the oven to 450°F.
2. Season the steaks with salt and pepper.
3. Wrap each steak snugly around the edges with 2 slices of bacon and secure the bacon with toothpicks.
4. Place a large skillet over medium-high heat and add the olive oil.
5. Pan sear the steaks for 4 minutes per side and transfer them to a baking sheet.
6. Roast the steaks until they reach your desired doneness, about 6 minutes for medium.
7. Remove the steaks from the oven and let them rest for 10 minutes.
8. Remove the toothpicks and serve.

A CLOSER LOOK Bacon has a bad reputation in many nutritionist circles because it can be very high in preservatives and sodium, depending on the brand and processing. Look for organic bacon with no additives, preferably from a reputable butcher.

PER SERVING Calories: 565; Fat: 49g; Protein: 28g; Carbs: 0g; Fiber: 0g; Net Carbs: 0g; Fat 78%/Protein 22%/Carbs 0%

CHEESEBURGER CASSEROLE

Serves 6 / Prep time: 10 minutes / Cook time: 40 minutes

Casseroles are the epitome of comfort food, and the no-fuss preparation is attractive for anyone who has a busy schedule to maintain. The favor of this dish will remind you of sizzling cheese-topped beef burgers right off the barbecue on a balmy summer evening. If you have leftovers, either enjoy them for lunch the next day or freeze them for up to 2 weeks.

1 pound 75% lean ground beef
½ cup chopped sweet onion
2 teaspoons minced garlic
1½ cups shredded aged Cheddar, divided
½ cup heavy (whipping) cream

1 large tomato, chopped
1 teaspoon minced fresh basil
¼ teaspoon sea salt
⅛ teaspoon freshly ground black pepper

1. Preheat the oven to 350°F.
2. Place a large skillet over medium-high heat and add the ground beef.
3. Brown the beef until cooked through, about 6 minutes, and spoon off any excess fat.
4. Stir in the onion and garlic and cook until the vegetables are tender, about 4 minutes.
5. Transfer the beef and vegetables to an 8-by-8-inch casserole dish.
6. In medium bowl, stir together 1 cup of shredded cheese and the heavy cream, tomato, basil, salt, and pepper until well combined.
7. Pour the cream mixture over the beef mixture and top the casserole with the remaining ½ cup of shredded cheese.
8. Bake until the casserole is bubbly and the cheese is melted and lightly browned, about 30 minutes.
9. Serve.

PER SERVING Calories: 410; Fat: 33g; Protein: 20g; Carbs: 3g; Fiber: 0g; Net Carbs: 3g; Fat 75%/Protein 22%/Carbs 3%

ITALIAN BEEF BURGERS

Serves 4 / Prep time: 10 minutes / Cook time: 12 minutes

KETO QUOTIENT

DAIRY FREE
GLUTEN FREE
UNDER 30 MINUTES

Sometimes it is more fun to plan the toppings on a burger than is to make the burger itself. You can top these juicy patties with whatever catches your imagination, such as bacon, avocado, homemade mayonnaise, or simple tomato slices—or all of the above and more. Tomatoes are a wonderful choice because they are very high in vitamins A, C, and K and a phytonutrient called lycopene, which can help prevent certain cancers and support a healthy cardiovascular system.

1 pound 75% lean ground beef

¼ cup ground almonds

2 tablespoons chopped fresh basil

1 teaspoon minced garlic

¼ teaspoon sea salt

1 tablespoon olive oil

1 tomato, cut into 4 thick slices

¼ sweet onion, sliced thinly

1. In a medium bowl, mix together the ground beef, ground almonds, basil, garlic, and salt until well mixed.

2. Form the beef mixture into four equal patties and flatten them to about ½ inch thick.

3. Place a large skillet on medium-high heat and add the olive oil.

4. Panfry the burgers until cooked through, flipping them once, about 12 minutes in total.

5. Pat away any excess grease with paper towels and serve the burgers with a slice of tomato and onion.

SUBSTITUTION TIP Ground lamb is a perfect choice if you do not want to use ground beef; just make sure the ground meat is not too lean. Try to get 70% lean or less so that your fat macros are not too low.

PER SERVING Calories: 441; Fat: 37g; Protein: 22g; Carbs: 4g; Fiber: 1g; Net Carbs: 3g; Fat 76%/Protein 21%/Carbs 3%

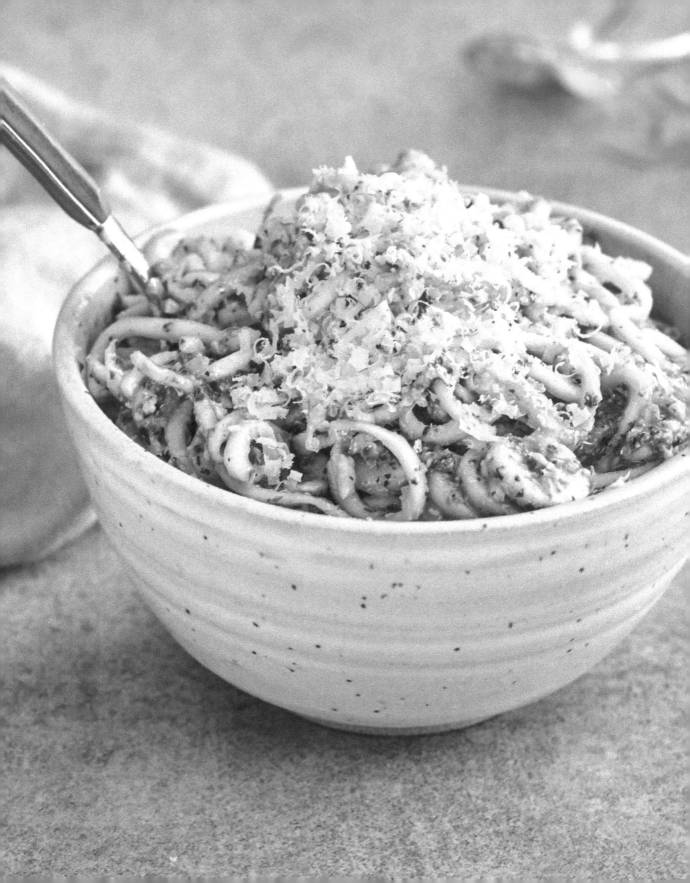

CHAPTER 7

VEGGIES & SIDES

◄ Pesto Zucchini Noodles, page 114

PORTOBELLO MUSHROOM PIZZA

Serves 4 / Prep time: 15 minutes / Cook time: 5 minutes

What would pizza be without gooey melted mozzarella? Mozzarella is produced using a method that spins the cheese from milk and then cuts it, called pasta filata. *Mozzarella is a good choice for the keto diet. It is high in fat (65 percent), contains about 32 percent protein, and has only 3 percent carbs.*

4 large portobello mushrooms, stems removed

¼ cup olive oil

1 teaspoon minced garlic

1 medium tomato, cut into 4 slices

2 teaspoons chopped fresh basil

1 cup shredded mozzarella cheese

1. Preheat the oven to broil. Line a baking sheet with aluminum foil and set aside.

2. In a small bowl, toss the mushroom caps with the olive oil until well coated. Use your fingertips to rub the oil in without breaking the mushrooms.

3. Place the mushrooms on the baking sheet gill-side down and broil the mushrooms until they are tender on the tops, about 2 minutes.

4. Flip the mushrooms over and broil 1 minute more.

5. Take the baking sheet out and spread the garlic over each mushroom, top each with a tomato slice, sprinkle with the basil, and top with the cheese.

6. Broil the mushrooms until the cheese is melted and bubbly, about 1 minute.

7. Serve.

PAIRS WELL WITH These pizzas pack a lot of flavor, so you'll need an assertive main course to share the plate with them. Some wonderful options could include Bacon-Wrapped Beef Tenderloin (page 101) or Sirloin with Blue Cheese Compound Butter (page 98). These juicy mushrooms make a tempting snack, as well.

PER SERVING Calories: 251; Fat: 20g; Protein: 14g; Carbs: 7g; Fiber: 3g; Net Carbs: 4g; Fat 71%/Protein 19%/Carbs 10%

GARLICKY GREEN BEANS

Serves 4 / Prep time: 10 minutes / Cook time: 10 minutes

KETO QUOTIENT

GLUTEN FREE
NUT FREE
VEGETARIAN
UNDER 30 MINUTES

Sizzling lightly caramelized green beans flavored generously with garlic are a perfect culinary storm of texture, color, and taste. You might find yourself whipping up a batch to eat as a snack instead of a side dish. Yellow wax beans or a combination of the two colors would also be a lovely choice if you want to vary the ingredients.

1 pound green beans, stemmed

2 tablespoons olive oil

1 teaspoon minced garlic

Sea salt

Freshly ground black pepper

¼ cup freshly grated Parmesan cheese

1. Preheat the oven to 425°F. Line a baking sheet with aluminum foil and set aside.

2. In a large bowl, toss together the green beans, olive oil, and garlic until well mixed.

3. Season the beans lightly with salt and pepper.

4. Spread the beans on the baking sheet and roast them until they are tender and lightly browned, stirring them once, about 10 minutes.

5. Serve topped with the Parmesan cheese.

PAIRS WELL WITH Look for entrées with a quick cooking time so that your entire meal can be on the table in less than 30 minutes. Try tender Herb Butter Scallops (page 75) or Pan-Seared Halibut with Citrus Butter Sauce (page 76) for a lovely, speedy meal.

PER SERVING Calories: 104; Fat: 9g; Protein: 4g; Carbs: 2g; Fiber: 1g; Net Carbs: 1g; Fat 77%/Protein 15%/Carbs 8%

SAUTÉED ASPARAGUS WITH WALNUTS

Serves 4 / Prep time: 10 minutes / Cook time: 5 minutes

If you are a foodie, you probably wait with anticipation for spring and the slender elegant asparagus spears that come into season at that time. Asparagus is a good choice for keto followers because although this veggie contains carbs, it is also very high in fiber, which creates a low net carb result. Asparagus is an antioxidant and anti-inflammatory, so it is excellent for eye health, helps fight cancers, and is wonderful for your heart.

1½ tablespoons olive oil
¾ pound asparagus, woody
  ends trimmed

Sea salt
Freshly ground pepper
¼ cup chopped walnuts

1. Place a large skillet over medium-high heat and add the olive oil.
2. Sauté the asparagus until the spears are tender and lightly browned, about 5 minutes.
3. Season the asparagus with salt and pepper.
4. Remove the skillet from the heat and toss the asparagus with the walnuts.
5. Serve.

PAIRS WELL WITH There are very few other ingredients that do not combine well with asparagus, so you have many delicious options for main dishes to serve with these tasty spears. Good choices to consider are Paprika Chicken (page 85) or Roasted Pork Loin with Grainy Mustard Sauce (page 93).

PER SERVING Calories: 124; Fat: 12g; Protein: 3g; Carbs: 4g; Fiber: 2g; Net Carbs: 2g; Fat 81%/Protein 9%/Carbs 10%

BRUSSELS SPROUTS CASSEROLE

Serves 8 / Prep time: 15 minutes / Cook time: 30 minutes

KETO QUOTIENT

GLUTEN FREE
NUT FREE

Brussels sprouts are often left in the produce section of the grocery store because they look complicated to cook. And if you have ever overcooked them, they produce an extremely unpleasant sulphur-like odor. You should rethink this nutritional powerhouse because they are delicious and have many health benefits. Brussels sprouts help fight cardiovascular disease and cancer, lower cholesterol levels, and can improve thyroid function. And they really are easy to cook well.

8 bacon slices

1 pound Brussels sprouts, blanched for 10 minutes and cut into quarters

1 cup shredded Swiss cheese, divided

¾ cup heavy (whipping) cream

1. Preheat the oven to 400°F.

2. Place a skillet over medium-high heat and cook the bacon until it is crispy, about 6 minutes.

3. Reserve 1 tablespoon of bacon fat to grease the casserole dish and roughly chop the cooked bacon.

4. Lightly oil a casserole dish with the reserved bacon fat and set aside.

5. In a medium bowl, toss the Brussels sprouts with the chopped bacon and ½ cup of cheese and transfer the mixture to the casserole dish.

6. Pour the heavy cream over the Brussels sprouts and top the casserole with the remaining ½ cup of cheese.

7. Bake until the cheese is melted and lightly browned and the vegetables are heated through, about 20 minutes.

8. Serve.

PAIRS WELL WITH This rich dish needs a simple entrée on the plate so that you don't feel too full at the end of the meal. Consider Italian Beef Burgers (page 103) or Rosemary-Garlic Lamb Racks (page 96).

PER SERVING Calories: 299; Fat: 11g; Protein: 12g; Carbs: 7g; Fiber: 3g; Net Carbs: 4g; Fat 77%/Protein 15%/Carbs 8%

CREAMED SPINACH

Serves 4 / Prep time: 10 minutes / Cook time: 30 minutes

Creamed vegetables, spinach in particular, have been around for several thousand years, although in the past several years, yogurt was often used in the sauce instead of heavy cream. The finished dish is comforting and perfect for large potluck events when you need to bring something to contribute. If you want to cut some of the calories from the recipe, swap out the heavy cream for evaporated milk, but keep in mind that also changes the keto macro.

1 tablespoon butter
½ sweet onion, very thinly sliced
4 cups spinach, stemmed and
  thoroughly washed
¾ cup heavy (whipping) cream

¼ cup Herbed Chicken Stock
  (page 141)
Pinch sea salt
Pinch freshly ground black pepper
Pinch ground nutmeg

1. In a large skillet over medium heat, add the butter.
2. Sauté the onion until it is lightly caramelized, about 5 minutes.
3. Stir in the spinach, heavy cream, chicken stock, salt, pepper, and nutmeg.
4. Sauté until the spinach is wilted, about 5 minutes.
5. Continue cooking the spinach until it is tender and the sauce is thickened, about 15 minutes.
6. Serve immediately.

PAIRS WELL WITH Adding some color to your meal highlights the simple presentation of this traditional side dish. Look to Roasted Salmon with Avocado Salsa (page 78) for some pizzazz or a subtler Stuffed Chicken Breasts (page 86).

PER SERVING Calories: 195; Fat: 20g; Protein: 3g; Carbs: 3g; Fiber: 2g; Net Carbs: 1g; Fat 88%/Protein 6%/Carbs 6%

CHEESY MASHED CAULIFLOWER

Serves 4 / Prep time: 15 minutes / Cook time: 5 minutes

KETO QUOTIENT

GLUTEN FREE
NUT FREE
VEGETARIAN
UNDER 30 MINUTES

Mashed potatoes might be one of the foods you miss when starting your keto experience, but take heart because this lower-carb version is pretty close to its fluffy counterpart. The cheese, cream, and butter add lots of flavor and a certain creamy feel to the mashed cauliflower, and create a wonderful base for other variations. Try mashed roasted garlic in your cauliflower mash for a truly sublime side dish.

1 head cauliflower, chopped roughly
½ cup shredded Cheddar cheese
¼ cup heavy (whipping) cream

2 tablespoons butter, at room temperature
Sea salt
Freshly ground black pepper

1. Place a large saucepan filled three-quarters full with water over high heat and bring to a boil.

2. Blanch the cauliflower until tender, about 5 minutes, and drain.

3. Transfer the cauliflower to a food processor and add the cheese, heavy cream, and butter. Purée until very creamy and whipped.

4. Season with salt and pepper.

5. Serve.

PAIRS WELL WITH Creamy mashed vegetables seem to call out for delectable sauces to spoon over them. Two of the best come with the Garlic-Braised Short Ribs (page 100) and Coconut Chicken (page 87).

PER SERVING Calories: 183; Fat: 15g; Protein: 8g; Carbs: 6g; Fiber: 2g; Net Carbs: 4g; Fat 75%/Protein 14%/Carbs 11%

SAUTÉED CRISPY ZUCCHINI

KETO QUOTIENT

GLUTEN FREE
NUT FREE
VEGETARIAN
UNDER 30 MINUTES

Serves 4 / Prep time: 15 minutes/ Cook time: 10 minutes

Anyone who has eaten a grilled cheese sandwich or picked the crispy edges off of a lasagna knows how incredible these cheesy bits taste. That rich golden crisp cheese is what you end up with on your sautéed zucchini when you prepare this recipe. The trick is to let the ingredients sit in the skillet after you add the cheese so it has the chance to melt and lightly caramelize before stirring.

2 tablespoons butter
4 zucchini, cut into
¼-inch-thick rounds

½ cup freshly grated Parmesan
cheese
Freshly ground black pepper

1. Place a large skillet over medium-high heat and melt the butter.
2. Add the zucchini and sauté until tender and lightly browned, about 5 minutes.
3. Spread the zucchini evenly in the skillet and sprinkle the Parmesan cheese over the vegetables.
4. Cook without stirring until the Parmesan cheese is melted and crispy where it touches the skillet, about 5 minutes.
5. Serve.

PAIR WELL WITH The crispy bits of cheese are perfect with the lightly caramelized vegetables and are an attractive pairing with most entrées. Paprika Chicken (page 85) or Lamb Leg with Sun-Dried Tomato Pesto (page 97) would be delicious with this recipe.

PER SERVING Calories: 94; Fat: 8g; Protein: 4g; Carbs: 1g; Fiber: 0g;
Net Carbs: 1g; Fat 76%/Protein 20%/Carbs 4%

MUSHROOMS WITH CAMEMBERT

Serves 4 / Prep time: 5 minutes / Cook time: 15 minutes

Mushrooms have an interesting, almost meaty texture, and they tend to soak up all the flavorings in a recipe. Mushrooms are very high in vitamin D, the only vegetable source of this nutrient, and are an excellent source of potassium and selenium. Mushrooms can help reduce your cravings for sweet foods and help prevent spikes in blood sugar that can cause overeating.

2 tablespoons butter

2 teaspoons minced garlic

1 pound button mushrooms, halved

4 ounces Camembert cheese, diced

Freshly ground black pepper

1. Place a large skillet over medium-high heat and melt the butter.

2. Sauté the garlic until translucent, about 3 minutes.

3. Sauté the mushrooms until tender, about 10 minutes.

4. Stir in the cheese and sauté until melted, about 2 minutes.

5. Season with pepper and serve.

PAIRS WELL WITH A somewhat elegant dish like these cheesy mushrooms deserves to be matched with a gorgeous culinary partner. Very good choices include the Nut-Stuffed Pork Chops (page 92) or Lamb Chops with Kalamata Tapenade (page 94).

PER SERVING Calories: 161; Fat: 13g; Protein: 9g; Carbs: 4g; Fiber: 1g; Net Carbs: 3g; Fat 70%/Protein 21%/Carbs 9%

PESTO ZUCCHINI NOODLES

Serves 4 / Prep time: 15 minutes

The pesto recommended for this pretty side is the kale version found on page 131. Kale is touted as a super food for good reason, since this leafy green is very high in fiber, calcium, and vitamins A, C, and K. Kale helps lower cholesterol and reduces your risk for several cancers as well as boosting the immune system and detoxing the body.

4 small zucchini, ends trimmed
¾ cup Herb Kale Pesto (page 133)

¼ cup grated or shredded Parmesan cheese

1. Use a spiralizer or peeler to cut the zucchini into "noodles" and place them in a medium bowl.
2. Add the pesto and the Parmesan cheese and toss to coat.
3. Serve.

PAIRS WELL WITH This is a light side dish that is ready in an instant but packs a great deal of flavor. Try a simply flavored entrée to complement the freshness of the zucchini noodles, such as Pan-Seared Halibut with Citrus Butter Sauce (page 76) or Rosemary-Garlic Lamb Racks (page 96).

PER SERVING Calories: 93; Fat: 8g; Protein: 4g; Carbs: 2g; Fiber: 0g; Net Carbs: 2g; Fat 70%/Protein 15%/Carbs 8%

GOLDEN ROSTI

Serves 8 / Prep time: 15 minutes / Cook time: 15 minutes

KETO QUOTIENT

GLUTEN FREE
NUT FREE
UNDER 30 MINUTES

Celeriac has a parsley-like flavor and fresh scent under its gnarled skin. This root vegetable is a good source of phosphorus, potassium, fiber, iron, and vitamin C. It is also very low in calories, about 40 calories per cup.

8 bacon slices, chopped

1 cup shredded acorn squash

1 cup shredded raw celeriac

2 tablespoons grated or shredded Parmesan cheese

2 teaspoons minced garlic

1 teaspoon chopped fresh thyme

Sea salt

Freshly ground black pepper

2 tablespoons butter

1. In a large skillet over medium-high heat, cook the bacon until crispy, about 5 minutes.

2. While the bacon is cooking, in a large bowl, mix together the squash, celeriac, Parmesan cheese, garlic, and thyme. Season the mixture generously with salt and pepper, and set aside.

3. Remove the cooked bacon with a slotted spoon to the rosti mixture and stir to incorporate.

4. Remove all but 2 tablespoons of bacon fat from the skillet and add the butter.

5. Reduce the heat to medium-low and transfer the rosti mixture to the skillet and spread it out evenly to form a large round patty about 1 inch thick.

6. Cook until the bottom of the rosti is golden brown and crisp, about 5 minutes.

7. Flip the rosti over and cook until the other side is crispy and the middle is cooked through, about 5 minutes more.

8. Remove the skillet from the heat and cut the rosti into 8 pieces.

9. Serve.

PAIRS WELL WITH Rosti is great with comfort food. Serve with Turkey Meatloaf (page 88) or Lamb Leg with Sun-Dried Tomato Pesto (page 97).

PER SERVING Calories: 171; Fat: 15g; Protein: 5g; Carbs: 3g; Fiber: 0g; Net Carbs: 3g; Fat 81%/Protein 12%/Carbs 7%

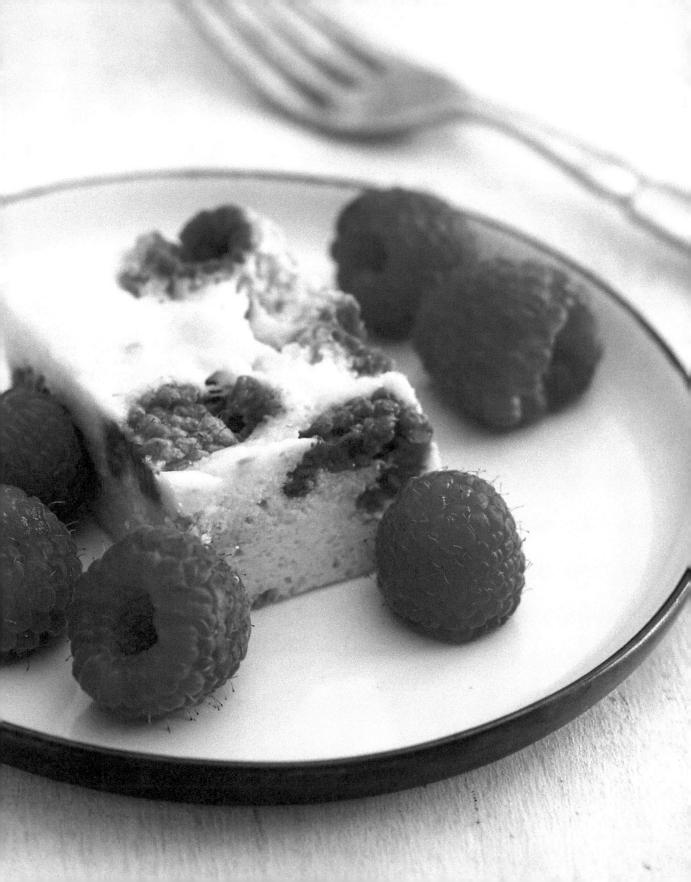

DESSERTS

◄ Raspberry Cheesecake, page 126

PUMPKIN SPICE FAT BOMBS

Makes 16 fat bombs / Prep time: 10 minutes, plus 1 hour chilling time

Pumpkin is a natural choice for desserts, especially those that also include warm spices reminiscent of holiday pumpkin pie. Like its vegetable counterpart, carrots, the bright orange flesh of pumpkin indicates it is a stellar source of beta-carotene. Pumpkin is also very high in vitamins A and C as well as potassium, making this pretty ingredient perfect for flushing toxins from your body and fighting cancer.

½ cup butter, at room temperature

½ cup cream cheese, at room temperature

⅓ cup pure pumpkin purée

3 tablespoons chopped almonds

4 drops liquid stevia

½ teaspoon ground cinnamon

¼ teaspoon ground nutmeg

1. Line an 8-by-8-inch pan with parchment paper and set aside.

2. In a small bowl, whisk together the butter and cream cheese until very smooth.

3. Add the pumpkin purée and whisk until blended.

4. Stir in the almonds, stevia, cinnamon, and nutmeg.

5. Spoon the pumpkin mixture into the pan. Use a spatula or the back of a spoon to spread it evenly in the pan, then place it in the freezer for about 1 hour.

6. Cut into 16 pieces and store the fat bombs in a tightly sealed container in the freezer until ready to serve.

PER SERVING (1 FAT BOMB) Calories: 87; Fat: 9g; Protein: 1g; Carbs: 1g; Fiber: 0g; Net Carbs: 1g; Fat 90%/Protein 5%/Carbs 5%

CREAMY BANANA FAT BOMBS

Makes 12 fat bombs / Prep time: 10 minutes, plus 1 hour chilling time

Banana-flavored desserts are a strange combination of exotic and comforting, as well as undeniably delicious. Fat bombs fall into savory or sweet categories, with these being on the sweeter side, but you can reduce the amount of sweetener if you want a less dessert-like experience. A sprinkling of shredded toasted coconut would top off these fat bombs beautifully.

1¼ cups cream cheese, at room temperature

¾ cup heavy (whipping) cream

1 tablespoon pure banana extract

6 drops liquid stevia

1. Line a baking sheet with parchment paper and set aside.

2. In a medium bowl, beat together the cream cheese, heavy cream, banana extract, and stevia until smooth and very thick, about 5 minutes.

3. Gently spoon the mixture onto the baking sheet in mounds, leaving some space between each mound, and place the baking sheet in the refrigerator until firm, about 1 hour.

4. Store the fat bombs in an airtight container in the refrigerator for up to 1 week.

A CLOSER LOOK Banana extract does have alcohol in it, but there is very little in each fat bomb, so they can be used on occasion for treats. You can use vanilla extract or almond extract, as well.

PER SERVING Calories: 134; Fat: 12g; Protein: 3g; Carbs: 1g; Fiber: 0g; Net Carbs: 1g; Fat 88%/Protein 9%/Carbs 3%

BLUEBERRY FAT BOMBS

Makes 12 fat bombs / Prep time: 10 minutes, plus 3 hours chilling time

The color of these fat bombs is a distinct blue, which you might find startling because very few foods are blue. Frozen unsweetened berries will work if fresh are not available or in season: Just thaw the frozen fruit first. If your area has wild blueberries, utilize these smaller berries because they have a significantly higher level of antioxidants than cultivated blueberries.

½ cup coconut oil, at room
  temperature
½ cup cream cheese, at room
  temperature

½ cup blueberries, mashed
  with a fork
6 drops liquid stevia
Pinch ground nutmeg

1. Line a mini muffin tin with paper liners and set aside.
2. In a medium bowl, stir together the coconut oil and cream cheese until well blended.
3. Stir in the blueberries, stevia, and nutmeg until combined.
4. Divide the blueberry mixture into the muffin cups and place the tray in the freezer until set, about 3 hours.
5. Place the fat bombs in an airtight container and store in the freezer until you wish to eat them.

PER SERVING Calories: 115; Fat: 12g; Protein: 1g; Carbs: 1g; Fiber: 0g; Net Carbs: 1g; Fat 94%/Protein 3%/Carbs 3%

SPICED-CHOCOLATE FAT BOMBS

KETO QUOTIENT

DAIRY FREE
GLUTEN FREE
VEGETARIAN

Makes 12 fat bombs / Prep time: 10 minutes, plus 15 minutes chilling time /
Cook time: 4 minutes

Good-quality cocoa powder is an acceptable ingredient on the keto diet, which means you can still enjoy a chocolate dessert and snack when you need a fix. Dark chocolate such as cocoa is very high in manganese, magnesium, copper, iron, and fiber as well as antioxidants, which fight free radicals in the body. Dark chocolate has been found to help lower blood pressure, reduce cholesterol, and improve cognitive function.

¾ cup coconut oil

¼ cup cocoa powder

¼ cup almond butter

⅛ teaspoon chili powder

3 drops liquid stevia

1. Line a mini muffin tin with paper liners and set aside.

2. Put a small saucepan over low heat and add the coconut oil, cocoa powder, almond butter, chili powder, and stevia.

3. Heat until the coconut oil is melted, then whisk to blend.

4. Spoon the mixture into the muffin cups and place the tin in the refrigerator until the bombs are firm, about 15 minutes.

5. Transfer the cups to an airtight container and store the fat bombs in the freezer until you want to serve them.

PER SERVING (1 FAT BOMB) Calories: 117; Fat: 12g; Protein: 2g; Carbs: 2g; Fiber: 0g; Net Carbs: 2g; Fat 92%/Protein 4%/Carbs 4%

CHOCOLATE-COCONUT TREATS

Makes 16 treats / Prep time: 10 minutes, plus 30 minutes chilling time /
Cook time: 3 minutes

Chocolate and coconut is a flawless combination often found in candy bars and many desserts. If you want a more elegant presentation, omit the coconut in step 3 and roll the semihardened chocolate mixture into balls instead of spreading it in a pan. Then roll the balls in the shredded coconut and place the treats in the freezer to firm up completely.

⅓ cup coconut oil

¼ cup unsweetened cocoa powder

4 drops liquid stevia

Pinch sea salt

¼ cup shredded unsweetened
  coconut

1. Line a 6-by-6-inch baking dish with parchment paper and set aside.
2. In a small saucepan over low heat, stir together the coconut oil, cocoa, stevia, and salt for about 3 minutes.
3. Stir in the coconut and press the mixture into the baking dish.
4. Place the baking dish in the refrigerator until the mixture is hard, about 30 minutes.
5. Cut into 16 pieces and store the treats in an airtight container in a cool place.

PREP TIP For a more finished look, you can spoon the hot mixture into candy molds instead of a baking dish. Pop the molds in the refrigerator for 30 minutes or until firm and pop the treats out into a container.

PER SERVING (1 TREAT) Calories: 43; Fat: 5g; Protein: 1g; Carbs: 1g; Fiber: 0g; Net Carbs: 1g; Fat 88%/Protein 6%/Carbs 6%

ALMOND BUTTER FUDGE

KETO QUOTIENT

GLUTEN FREE
VEGETARIAN

Makes 36 pieces / Prep time: 10 minutes, plus 2 hours chilling time

Fudge should be smooth and dense with no grittiness or graininess. Since you won't be using granulated sugar for this treat, the chances of getting the wrong texture are greatly reduced. Almond butter is a stellar source of protein, vitamin E, iron, manganese, and fiber. If you are not a fan of this nut butter, peanut butter or cashew butter would also be delicious and create the same tempting results.

1 cup coconut oil, at room temperature

1 cup almond butter

¼ cup heavy (whipping) cream

10 drops liquid stevia

Pinch sea salt

1. Line a 6-by-6-inch baking dish with parchment paper and set aside.

2. In a medium bowl, whisk together the coconut oil, almond butter, heavy cream, stevia, and salt until very smooth.

3. Spoon the mixture into the baking dish and smooth the top with a spatula.

4. Place the dish in the refrigerator until the fudge is firm, about 2 hours.

5. Cut into 36 pieces and store the fudge in an airtight container in the freezer for up to 2 weeks.

PER SERVING (2 PIECES OF FUDGE) Calories: 204; Fat: 22g; Protein: 3g; Carbs: 3g; Fiber: 1g; Net Carbs: 2g; Fat 90%/Protein 5%/Carbs 5%

KETO QUOTIENT

GLUTEN FREE
VEGETARIAN

NUTTY SHORTBREAD COOKIES

Makes 18 cookies / Prep time: 10 minutes, plus 30 minutes chilling time /
Cook time: 10 minutes

Traditional shortbread has very few ingredients and is intensely buttery, slightly crumbly, and not too sweet. The nuts used here in place of flour create the desired texture and add a complex, pleasing flavor. These cookies will continue to cook on the baking sheets after you take them out of the oven, so don't forget to transfer them to wire racks quickly to avoid overbrowning.

½ cup butter, at room temperature, plus additional for greasing the baking sheet

½ cup granulated sweetener

1 teaspoon alcohol-free pure vanilla extract

1½ cups almond flour

½ cup ground hazelnuts

Pinch sea salt

1. In a medium bowl, cream together the butter, sweetener, and vanilla until well blended.

2. Stir in the almond flour, ground hazelnuts, and salt until a firm dough is formed.

3. Roll the dough into a 2-inch cylinder and wrap it in plastic wrap. Place the dough in the refrigerator for at least 30 minutes until firm.

4. Preheat the oven to 350°F. Line a baking sheet with parchment paper and lightly grease the paper with butter; set aside.

5. Unwrap the chilled cylinder, slice the dough into 18 cookies, and place the cookies on the baking sheet.

6. Bake the cookies until firm and lightly browned, about 10 minutes.

7. Allow the cookies to cool on the baking sheet for 5 minutes and then transfer them to a wire rack to cool completely.

PREP TIP Process less expensive whole nuts in a food processor or blender rather than paying for a preground product. Make sure you don't process the nuts in the appliance too long or you'll end up with nut butter.

PER SERVING (1 COOKIE) Calories: 105; Fat: 10g; Protein: 3g; Carbs: 2g; Fiber: 1g; Net Carbs: 1g; Fat 85%/Protein 9%/Carbs 6%

VANILLA-ALMOND ICE POPS

KETO QUOTIENT

GLUTEN FREE
VEGETARIAN

Makes 8 ice pops / Prep time: 10 minutes, plus 4 hours freezing time /
Cook time: 5 minutes

In childhood, nothing was better than a sweet treat on a hot summer day. This is a more elegant ice pop that can be enjoyed after a leisurely barbecue with friends. It features simple vanilla and coconut flavoring, which can be enhanced with cut fruit if you want a little more texture to the pop. Use inexpensive ice pop molds; they are easily found for a few dollars in most stores.

2 cups almond milk

1 cup heavy (whipping) cream

1 vanilla bean, halved lengthwise

1 cup shredded unsweetened coconut

1. Place a medium saucepan over medium heat and add the almond milk, heavy cream, and vanilla bean.

2. Bring the liquid to a simmer and reduce the heat to low. Continue to simmer for 5 minutes.

3. Remove the saucepan from the heat and let the liquid cool.

4. Take the vanilla bean out of the liquid and use a knife to scrape the seeds out of the bean into the liquid.

5. Stir in the coconut and divide the liquid between the ice pop molds.

6. Freeze until solid, about 4 hours, and enjoy.

PER SERVING (1 ICE POP) Calories: 166; Fat: 15g; Protein: 3g; Carbs: 4g;
Fiber: 2g; Net Carbs: 2g; Fat 81%/Protein 9%/Carbs 10%

RASPBERRY CHEESECAKE

Serves 12 / Prep time: 10 minutes / Cook time: 25 to 30 minutes

Cheesecake is a sublime dessert experience: tart, sweet, and infinitely velvety on the tongue. This is a crust-free cheesecake featuring plump ripe raspberries and a distinct vanilla undertone. You can use any type of berry, sliced peaches or plums, or even a tablespoon of cocoa powder to create gorgeous variations. Your imagination is the limit when you have a perfect cheesecake base to use in your experiments.

⅔ cup coconut oil, melted

½ cup cream cheese,
   at room temperature

6 eggs

3 tablespoons granulated
   sweetener

1 teaspoon alcohol-free pure
   vanilla extract

½ teaspoon baking powder

¾ cup raspberries

1. Preheat the oven to 350°F. Line an 8-by-8-inch baking dish with parchment paper and set aside.

2. In a large bowl, beat together the coconut oil and cream cheese until smooth.

3. Beat in the eggs, scraping down the sides of the bowl at least once.

4. Beat in the sweetener, vanilla, and baking powder until smooth.

5. Spoon the batter into the baking dish and use a spatula to smooth out the top. Scatter the raspberries on top.

6. Bake until the center is firm, about 25 to 30 minutes.

7. Allow the cheesecake to cool completely before cutting into 12 squares.

SUBSTITUTION TIP Any type of berry is delicious in this luscious treat, such as blueberries, strawberries, or blackberries. Whenever possible for your recipes, use seasonal local fruit for the best flavor and color.

PER SERVING (1 SQUARE) Calories: 176; Fat: 18g; Protein: 6g; Carbs: 3g; Fiber: 1g; Net Carbs: 2g; Fat 85%/Protein 11%/Carbs 4%

PEANUT BUTTER MOUSSE

Serves 4 / Prep time: 10 minutes, plus 30 minutes chilling time

Peanut butter is always a handy, delicious sandwich spread, but it is used in many types of dishes all over the world, and is very healthy. Eating peanut butter, even in this scrumptious dessert, can reduce your risk of cancer and heart disease, and help lower cholesterol levels. Natural peanut butter is very high in unsaturated fats, protein, fiber, and folate.

1 cup heavy (whipping) cream
¼ cup natural peanut butter

1 teaspoon alcohol-free pure
  vanilla extract
4 drops liquid stevia

1. In a medium bowl, beat together the heavy cream, peanut butter, vanilla, and stevia until firm peaks form, about 5 minutes.

2. Spoon the mousse into 4 bowls and place in the refrigerator to chill for 30 minutes.

3. Serve.

PER SERVING Calories: 280; Fat: 28g; Protein: 6g; Carbs: 4g; Fiber: 1g; Net Carbs: 3g; Fat 83%/Protein 10%/Carbs 7%

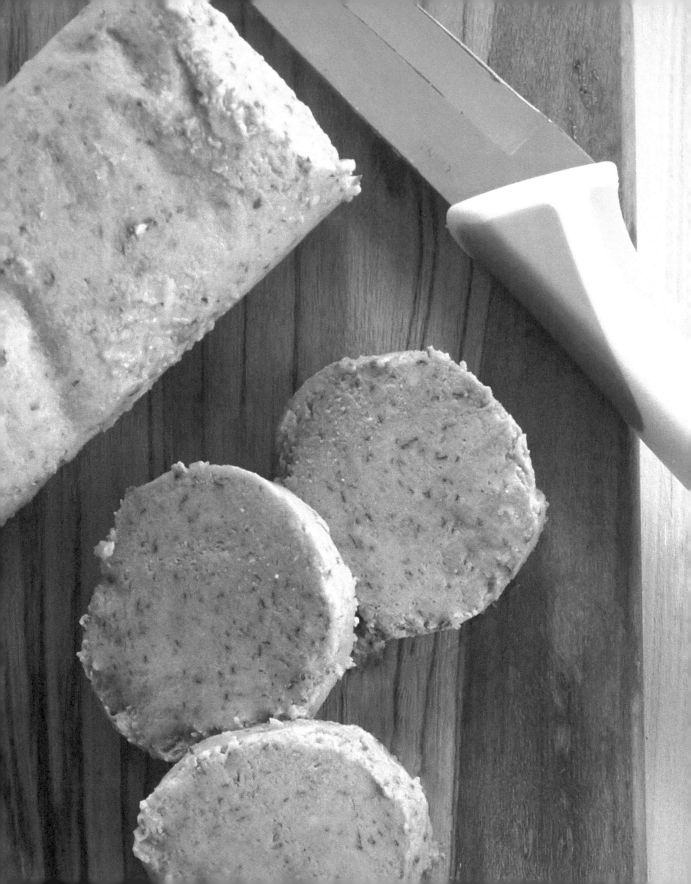

CHAPTER 9
STAPLES

◄ Avocado-Herb Compound Butter, page 130

AVOCADO-HERB COMPOUND BUTTER

Makes 2 cups / Prep time: 25 minutes, plus 4 hours chilling time

Avocado shows up a fair bit in keto recipes because it is a spectacular source of monounsaturated fats, oleic acid, and omega-3 fatty acids. This high-fat profile makes reaching your keto macros easier and can increase absorption of beta-carotene in other ingredients by as much as 400 percent. Avocado is also high in fiber and lutein.

¼ cup butter, at room temperature
1 avocado, peeled, pitted, and cut
  into quarters
Juice of ½ lemon
2 teaspoons chopped cilantro

1 teaspoon chopped fresh basil
1 teaspoon minced garlic
Sea salt
Freshly ground black pepper

1. Place the butter, avocado, lemon juice, cilantro, basil, and garlic in a food processor and process until smooth.
2. Season the butter with salt and pepper.
3. Transfer the mixture to a sheet of parchment paper and shape it into a log.
4. Place the parchment butter log in the refrigerator until it is firm, about 4 hours.
5. Serve slices of this butter with fish or chicken.
6. Store unused butter wrapped tightly in the freezer for up to 1 week.

PREP TIP The best avocados for this butter are ripe, soft fruit. Place unripe avocados in a paper bag for a few days with an apple or banana to speed up the ripening process.

PER SERVING (1 TABLESPOON) Calories: 22; Fat: 2g; Protein: 0g; Carbs: 1g; Fiber: 0g; Net Carbs: 1g; Fat 86%/Protein 3%/Carbs 11%

STRAWBERRY BUTTER

Makes 3 cups / Prep time: 25 minutes

KETO QUOTIENT

DAIRY FREE
GLUTEN FREE
NUT FREE
VEGETARIAN
UNDER 30 MINUTES

If you have ever picked your own strawberries, you will remember the heady sweet fragrance of ripe berries in the field and intense flavor of a berry warm from the sun. Strawberries are best picked organic or purchased organic because they top the Dirty Dozen list of pesticide-contaminated produce put out by the Environmental Working Group. If you cannot find organic berries, make sure you wash your fruit thoroughly to limit your exposure.

2 cups shredded unsweetened coconut

1 tablespoon coconut oil

¾ cup fresh strawberries

½ tablespoon freshly squeezed lemon juice

1 teaspoon alcohol-free pure vanilla extract

1. Put the coconut in a food processor and purée it until it is buttery and smooth, about 15 minutes.

2. Add the coconut oil, strawberries, lemon juice, and vanilla to the coconut butter and process until very smooth, scraping down the sides of the bowl.

3. Pass the butter through a fine sieve to remove the strawberry seeds, using the back of a spoon to press the butter through.

4. Store the strawberry butter in an airtight container in the refrigerator for up to 2 weeks.

5. Serve chicken or fish with a spoon of this butter on top.

PER SERVING (1 TABLESPOON) Calories: 23; Fat: 2g; Protein: 0g; Carbs: 1g; Fiber: 0g; Net Carbs: 1g; Fat 80%/Protein 5%/Carbs 15%

KETO QUOTIENT

DAIRY FREE
GLUTEN FREE
NUT FREE
VEGETARIAN
UNDER 30 MINUTES

HERBED BALSAMIC DRESSING

Makes 1 cup / Prep time: 4 minutes

Having a foolproof salad dressing recipe you can whip up on a moment's notice is a cook's essential. Vinaigrettes are not complicated, but you do need the correct ratios to create emulsification between the acid and oil. Balsamic vinegar adds a pleasing sweetness to this dressing, and since a little goes a long way, you won't be getting too many carbs from the vinegar.

1 cup extra-virgin olive oil
¼ cup balsamic vinegar
2 tablespoons chopped
  fresh oregano

1 teaspoon chopped fresh basil
1 teaspoon minced garlic
Sea salt
Freshly ground black pepper

1. Whisk the olive oil and vinegar in a small bowl until emulsified, about 3 minutes.

2. Whisk in the oregano, basil, and garlic until well combined, about 1 minute.

3. Season the dressing with salt and pepper.

4. Transfer the dressing to an airtight container, and store it in the refrigerator for up to 1 week. Give the dressing a vigorous shake before using it.

PER SERVING (1 TABLESPOON) Calories: 83; Fat: 9g; Protein: 0g; Carbs: 0g; Fiber: 0g; Net Carbs: 0g; Fat 100%/Protein 0%/Carbs 0%

HERB-KALE PESTO

Makes 1½ cups / Prep time: 15 minutes

KETO QUOTIENT

DAIRY FREE
GLUTEN FREE
NUT FREE
VEGETARIAN
UNDER 30 MINUTES

Nutritional yeast adds a lovely, almost cheesy taste to this pesto as well as a hearty amount of protein and fiber. Nutritional yeast is also a fabulous source of vitamin B_{12}, which is one of the most prevalent nutritional deficiencies in the world. Vitamin B_{12} is crucial for many metabolic functions and for help in maintaining both a healthy cardiovascular system and nervous system.

1 cup chopped kale

1 cup fresh basil leaves

3 garlic cloves

2 teaspoons nutritional yeast

¼ cup extra-virgin olive oil

1. Place the kale, basil, garlic, and yeast in a food processor and pulse until the mixture is finely chopped, about 3 minutes.
2. With the food processor running, drizzle the olive oil into the pesto until a thick paste forms, scraping down the sides of the bowl at least once.
3. Add a little water if the pesto is too thick.
4. Store the pesto in an airtight container in the refrigerator for up to 1 week.

SUBSTITUTION TIP Try spinach or any other dark leafy green in place of the kale for interesting variations. You can also use any of an assortment of different herbs in the same quantity as the basil in this recipe.

PER SERVING (2 TABLESPOONS) Calories: 44; Fat: 4g; Protein: 1g; Carbs: 1g; Fiber: 0g; Net Carbs: 1g; Fat 82%/Protein 9%/Carbs 9%

HOLLANDAISE

Makes 2 cups / Prep time: 20 minutes /
Cook time: 10 minutes, plus 15 minutes cooling time

You might think this sauce looks like a great deal of work, and you wouldn't be entirely wrong, but the luscious spoon-coating creation at the end of the process is more than worth the effort. Hollandaise does not keep longer than about 2 hours and only that long if the temperature in your kitchen is not too hot, so don't make more than you can use in one meal. Try adding some chopped tarragon to the hollandaise if you want to make a béarnaise sauce instead.

1½ cups unsalted butter
4 large egg yolks
2 teaspoons cold water

Juice of 1 small lemon,
    about 4 teaspoons
Pinch sea salt

1. Place a medium heavy-bottomed saucepan over very low heat and melt the butter.
2. Remove the saucepan from the heat and let the melted butter stand for 5 minutes.
3. Carefully skim the foam from the top of the melted butter.
4. Very slowly pour the clarified part of the butter (it should be a clear yellow color) into a container, leaving the milky solids in the bottom of the saucepan.
5. Discard the milky solids and let the clarified butter cool in the container until it is just warm, about 15 minutes.
6. Put a medium saucepan with about 3 inches of water in it over medium heat until the water simmers gently.
7. In a large stainless steel bowl, add the egg yolks and 2 teaspoons of cold water and whisk them until they are foamy and light, about 3 minutes.
8. Add 3 or 4 drops of the lemon juice to the yolks and whisk for about 1 minute.

9. Place the bowl onto the mouth of the saucepan, making sure the bottom of the bowl does not touch the simmering water.

10. Whisk the yolks until they thicken a little, about 1 to 2 minutes, then remove the bowl from the simmering water.

11. In a very thin stream, add the clarified butter to the yolk mixture, whisking continuously, until you have used up all the butter and your sauce is thick and smooth. If you add the butter too quickly, the sauce will break.

12. Whisk in the remaining lemon juice and the salt.

13. This sauce should be used right away or held for only about 1 hour. Throw away any unused sauce.

PER SERVING (1 TABLESPOON) Calories: 173; Fat: 17g; Protein: 5g; Carbs: 1g; Fiber: 0g; Net Carbs: 1g; Fat 86%/Protein 11%/Carbs 3%

GREEN BASIL DRESSING

Makes 1 cup / Prep time: 10 minutes

Basil has a unique licorice-like taste and delicate deep green leaves that create a wonderful dressing for a summer salad. This herb is a very effective antibacterial, which means bacteria growth is almost impossible in this dressing. Basil is very high in vitamin K, copper, flavonoids, and manganese. Grow your own in terra cotta pots on your patio or windowsill so that you always have fresh basil handy for your cooking needs.

1 avocado, peeled and pitted
¼ cup sour cream
¼ cup extra-virgin olive oil
¼ cup chopped fresh basil

1 tablespoon freshly squeezed
  lime juice
1 teaspoon minced garlic
Sea salt
Freshly ground black pepper

1. Place the avocado, sour cream, olive oil, basil, lime juice, and garlic in a food processor and pulse until smooth, scraping down the sides of the bowl once during processing.

2. Season the dressing with salt and pepper.

3. Keep the dressing in an airtight container in the refrigerator for 1 to 2 weeks.

PER SERVING (1 TABLESPOON) Calories: 173; Fat: 17g; Protein: 5g; Carbs: 1g; Fiber: 0g; Net Carbs: 1g; Fat 86%/Protein 11%/Carbs 3%

CREAMY MAYONNAISE

KETO QUOTIENT

DAIRY FREE
GLUTEN FREE
NUT FREE
VEGETARIAN
UNDER 30 MINUTES

Makes 4 cups / Prep time: 10 minutes

Homemade mayonnaise is a truly decadent condiment, and you can control the ingredients that go into the recipe. It's not difficult to make, especially with an immersion blender or food processor, but whisking up a batch by hand can be satisfying. It is fun to watch the ingredients emulsify before your eyes. Keep the mayonnaise in the refrigerator in an airtight container for up to 4 days.

2 large eggs

2 tablespoons Dijon mustard

1½ cups extra-virgin olive oil

¼ cup freshly squeezed lemon juice

Sea salt

Freshly ground black pepper

TO MAKE BY HAND

1. Whisk the eggs and mustard together in a heavy, large bowl until very well combined, about 2 minutes.

2. Add the oil in a continuous thin stream, whisking constantly, until the mayonnaise is thick and completely emulsified.

3. Add the lemon juice and whisk until well blended.

4. Season with salt and pepper.

TO MAKE IN A FOOD PROCESSOR

1. Place the eggs and mustard in the processor bowl and blend until very smooth.

2. While the processor is running, slowly add the oil in a thin stream until the mayonnaise is thick and completely emulsified.

3. Add the lemon juice and process until smooth.

4. Season with salt and pepper.

PER SERVING (2 TABLESPOONS) Calories: 61; Fat: 7g; Protein: 0g; Carbs: 0g; Fiber: 0g; Net Carbs: 0g; Fat 97%/Protein 2%/Carbs 1%

RICH BEEF STOCK

Makes 8 to 10 cups / Prep time: 15 minutes /
Cook time: 12½ hours, plus 30 minutes cooling time

If you have never attempted beef stock before, you might be wondering where to find beef bones for this recipe. Beef bones are actually quite common in many grocery store meat sections, usually a little out of the way next to the tongues and kidneys, but they are often prepackaged and displayed. If your store does not have beef bones in the cooler or freezer, ask your butcher—there may be some in the back, or you can ask them to save the bones from the next meat order.

2 to 3 pounds beef bones
  (beef marrow, knuckle bones,
  ribs, and any other bones)
8 black peppercorns
5 thyme sprigs
3 garlic cloves, peeled and crushed
2 bay leaves

1 carrot, washed and chopped
  into 2-inch pieces
1 celery stalk, chopped into
  big chunks
½ onion, peeled and quartered
1 gallon water
1 teaspoon extra-virgin olive oil

1. Preheat the oven to 350°F.
2. Place the beef bones in a deep baking pan and roast them in the oven for about 30 minutes.
3. Transfer the roasted bones to a large stockpot and add the peppercorns, thyme, garlic, bay leaves, carrot, celery, and onion.
4. Add the water, making sure the bones are completely covered.
5. Place the pot on high heat and bring to a boil, then reduce the heat to low so that the stock gently simmers.
6. Check the stock every hour, at least for the first 3 hours, and skim off any foam that forms on the top.

7. Simmer for 12 hours in total and then remove the pot from the heat. Cool the stock for about 30 minutes.

8. Remove any large bones with tongs and strain the stock through a fine-mesh sieve. Discard the leftover vegetables and bones.

9. Pour the stock into containers with tight-fitting lids and cool the stock completely before storing it in the refrigerator for up to 5 days or in the freezer for up to 2 months.

PER SERVING (1 CUP) Calories: 65; Fat: 5g; Protein: 4g; Carbs: 1g; Fiber: 0g; Net Carbs: 1g; Fat 70%/Protein 25%/Carbs 5%

DAIRY FREE
GLUTEN FREE
NUT FREE
UNDER 30 MINUTES

TRADITIONAL CAESAR DRESSING

Makes 1½ cups / Prep time: 10 minutes, plus 10 minutes cooling time / Cook time: 5 minutes

Caesar dressing used to be a culinary production in high-caliber restaurants, with waiters in black ties mixing all the ingredients tableside in huge wooden bowls. This type of spectacle is no longer part of most dining experiences, but the dressing remains as one of the most popular choices. If you want an even more authentic Caesar dressing, add a tablespoon of anchovy paste along with the mustard and vinegar.

2 teaspoons minced garlic

4 large egg yolks

¼ cup wine vinegar

½ teaspoon dry mustard

Dash Worcestershire sauce

1 cup extra-virgin olive oil

¼ cup freshly squeezed lemon juice

Sea salt

Freshly ground black pepper

1. To a small saucepan, add the garlic, egg yolks, vinegar, mustard, and Worcestershire sauce and place over low heat.

2. Whisking constantly, cook the mixture until it thickens and is a little bubbly, about 5 minutes.

3. Remove from saucepan from the heat and let it stand for about 10 minutes to cool.

4. Transfer the egg mixture to a large stainless steel bowl. Whisking constantly, add the olive oil in a thin stream.

5. Whisk in the lemon juice and season the dressing with salt and pepper.

6. Transfer the dressing to an airtight container and keep in the refrigerator for up to 3 days.

A CLOSER LOOK If you have concerns about raw egg yolks, you can purchase pasteurized eggs in most large supermarket chains. They are found alongside regular and specialty eggs in the dairy section.

PER SERVING (2 TABLESPOONS) Calories: 180; Fat: 20g; Protein: 1g; Carbs: 1g; Fiber: 0g; Net Carbs: 1g; Fat 96%/Protein 2%/Carbs 2%

HERBED CHICKEN STOCK

DAIRY FREE
GLUTEN FREE
NUT FREE

Makes 8 cups / Prep time: 15 minutes /
Cook time: 12 hours, plus 30 minutes cooling time

Chicken stock works well with many veggies and herb flavors. However, try to always include onions—they contain quercetin, a flavonoid which remains in the stock after the solids are strained out. Quercetin can help prevent diabetes, fight cancer, and promote a very healthy cardiovascular system.

2 chicken carcasses (see Tip)

6 black peppercorns

4 thyme sprigs

3 bay leaves

2 celery stalks, cut into quarters

1 carrot, washed and chopped roughly

1 sweet onion, peeled and quartered

1 gallon cold water (enough to cover the carcasses and vegetables)

1. Place the chicken carcasses in a large stockpot with the peppercorns, thyme, bay leaves, celery, carrot, and onion.

2. Add the water, making sure the carcasses and vegetables are completely covered, and place the pot on high heat. Bring it to a boil and then reduce the heat to low and gently simmer, stirring every few hours, for 12 hours.

3. Remove the pot from the heat and let the stock cool for 30 minutes. Remove any large bones with tongs and then strain the stock through a fine-mesh sieve. Discard the solid bits.

4. Pour the stock into containers with tight-fitting lids and cool completely. Store in the refrigerator for up to 5 days, or freeze the stock for up to 3 months.

PREP TIP Chicken carcasses can be frozen in zip-top bags. When you have two or three, make this lovely stock by putting the frozen carcasses right in the pot.

PER SERVING (1 CUP) Calories: 73; Fat: 5g; Protein: 5g; Carbs: 2g; Fiber: 0g; Net Carbs: 2g; Fat 62%/Protein 27%/Carbs 11%

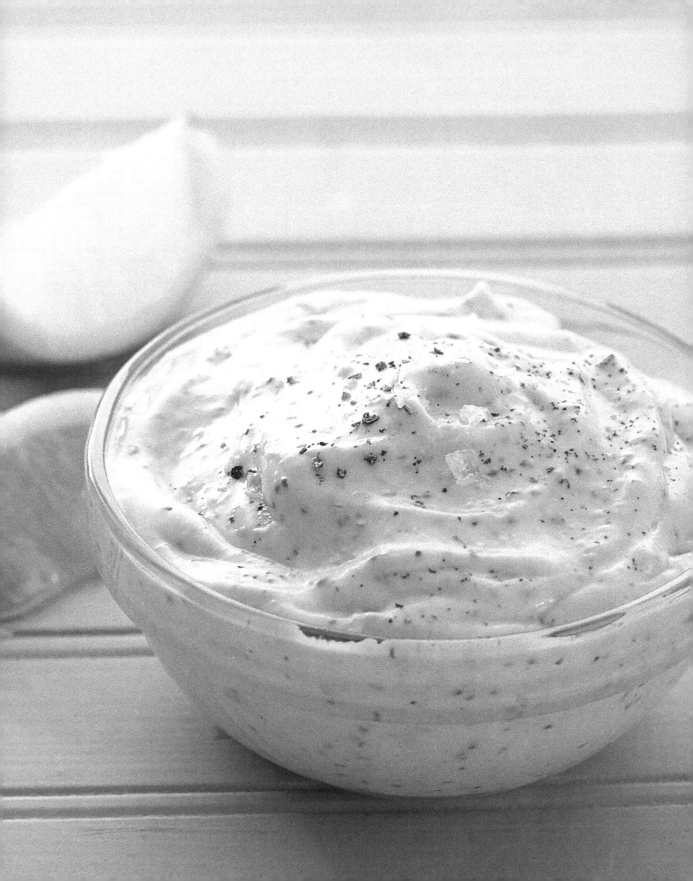

ADVICE FOR GOING OUT TO EAT

Getting rid of all culinary temptations is great for eating at home, but what happens when you go out to eat? Staying on a low-carb diet might seem difficult at first, but it can be easy with these few tips and a little bit of practice!

BREAKFAST

Skip the bagels, pancakes, Belgian waffles, French toast, or anything of the like. Opt for an omelet, or a few eggs with a side of sausage or ham. Skip the toast and hash browns.

LUNCH

Get a salad with lots of meat. Try a Cobb, chicken Caesar, or garden salad with chicken on top. Use plenty of olive oil and salt (electrolytes). You'll feel great afterward and have plenty of energy to last you until dinner. Carbs are why people get sleepy after lunch. Don't be a victim!

DINNER

When ordering a burger, ask to have it wrapped in lettuce. If they're unable to do that, just ask for no bun. If they bring the bun, take the patty and anything else off the bun and put it to the side. Skip the ketchup as well—it's full of sugar. Try mayo, mustard, red pepper sauce, sriracha, or any other low-carb sauce.

At Italian restaurants, skip the pasta and pizza, and order the protein-based dinners. Make sure to request salad or any other low-carb alternatives instead of the usual high-carb sides. If all else fails, just eat the topping off of the pizza and avoid the crust.

With Mexican cuisine, try to get your food in a bowl instead of in a burrito wrap or tortilla. Don't get rice or beans; instead, get extra sour cream and guacamole.

◄ Creamy Mayonnaise, page 137

SIDES

French fries, steak fries, mashed potatoes, baked potatoes, rice, beans, corn on the cob, banana bread, and any other high-carb sides can be replaced with salad, asparagus, broccoli, green beans, or other low-carb vegetables. Most restaurants have some sort of salad for you to choose from. Make sure to always ask and double-check with the waiter or staff.

DRINKS AND ALCOHOL

Instead of juice or soda, stick to water, tea, and coffee. Use heavy cream or half-and-half instead of milk.

In addition to fat, carbs, and protein, alcohol is also a macronutrient. It provides 7 calories per gram, the second most after fat, which provides 9 calories per gram. It is burned by the body before all the other macronutrients. If you drink too much alcohol, you will slow down your fat-burning process and impede your weight loss, if that is your goal.

If you're ordering alcohol, stay away from any cocktails, as they're all loaded with sugar. Dry or semidry wine has about 3 grams of carbs per glass, and low-carb beers like Michelob Ultra and Modelo have 3 to 4 grams of carbs per bottle. All pure spirits like vodka, Cognac, brandy, bourbon, whisky, rum, tequila, and gin are zero carbs. As always, drink in moderation, stay safe, and enjoy!

THE DIRTY DOZEN AND CLEAN FIFTEEN

A nonprofit and environmental watchdog organization called the Environmental Working Group (EWG) looks at data supplied by the US Department of Agriculture (USDA) and the Food and Drug Administration (FDA) about pesticide residues. Each year it compiles a list of the lowest and highest pesticide loads found in commercial crops. You can use these lists to decide which fruits and vegetables to buy organic to minimize your exposure to pesticides and which produce is considered safe enough to buy conventionally. This does not mean they are pesticide-free, though, so wash these fruits and vegetables thoroughly.

These lists change every year, so make sure you look up the most recent one before you fill your shopping cart. You'll find the most recent lists as well as a guide to pesticides in produce at EWG.org/FoodNews.

The Dirty Dozen

- Apples
- Celery
- Cherry tomatoes
- Cucumbers
- Grapes
- Nectarines (imported)
- Peaches
- Potatoes
- Snap peas (imported)
- Spinach
- Strawberries
- Sweet bell peppers

Kale/Collard greens & Hot peppers*

The Clean Fifteen

- Asparagus
- Avocados
- Cabbage
- Cantaloupes (domestic)
- Cauliflower
- Eggplants
- Grapefruits
- Kiwis
- Mangoes
- Onions
- Papayas
- Pineapples
- Sweet corn
- Sweet peas (frozen)
- Sweet potatoes

*In addition to the Dirty Dozen, the EWG added two produce items contaminated with highly toxic organo-phosphate insecticides.

MEASUREMENT CONVERSION TABLES

VOLUME EQUIVALENTS (LIQUID)

US STANDARD	US STANDARD (OUNCES)	METRIC (APPROXIMATE)
2 tablespoons	1 fl. oz.	30 mL
¼ cup	2 fl. oz.	60 mL
½ cup	4 fl. oz.	120 mL
1 cup	8 fl. oz.	240 mL
1½ cups	12 fl. oz.	355 mL
2 cups or 1 pint	16 fl. oz.	475 mL
4 cups or 1 quart	32 fl. oz.	1 L
1 gallon	128 fl. oz.	4 L

OVEN TEMPERATURES

FAHRENHEIT (F)	CELSIUS (C) (APPROXIMATE)
250°F	120°C
300°F	150°C
325°F	165°C
350°F	180°C
375°F	190°C
400°F	200°C
425°F	220°C
450°F	230°C

VOLUME EQUIVALENTS (DRY)

US STANDARD	METRIC (APPROXIMATE)
¼ teaspoon	1 mL
½ teaspoon	2 mL
1 teaspoon	5 mL
1 tablespoon	15 mL
¼ cup	59 mL
⅓ cup	79 mL
½ cup	118 mL
1 cup	235 mL

WEIGHT EQUIVALENTS

US STANDARD	METRIC (APPROXIMATE)
½ ounce	15 g
1 ounce	30 g
2 ounces	60 g
4 ounces	115 g
8 ounces	225 g
12 ounces	340 g
16 ounces or 1 pound	455 g

RESURCES

WEBSITES AND BLOGS

dietdoctor.com Diet Doctor is a low-carb-focused site that provides articles and recipes as well as instructional videos and support.

ketodietapp.com Keto Diet App is a keto-only blog and a great resource for science-backed articles and recipes. It also has an app for mobile devices which includes recipes, articles, meal planning, and progress tracking.

tasteaholics.com Tasteaholics is a keto-centric website and resource which provides science-backed articles and recipes.

authoritynutrition.com/ketogenic-diet-101 Authority Nutrition is not keto-centric, but it provides many science-backed articles and is a great resource overall.

alldayidreamaboutfood.com One of the oldest low-carb recipe blogs, with more recipes than any other low-carb blog.

reddit.com/r/keto A large community with hundreds of thousands of users, who discuss progress, share cravings, and support each other.

BOOKS

Moore, Jimmy, and Eric Westman. *Keto Clarity: Your Definitive Guide to the Benefits of a Low-Carb, High-Fat Diet.* (2014) Las Vegas, NV: Victory Belt Publishing.
A great read and further look into the science behind the keto diet and benefits from eating that diet.

Givens, Sara. *Ketogenic Diet Mistakes: You Wish You Knew.* (2014) Amazon Books. If you hit a weight-loss plateau or are running into any issues, this book can help you break through and reach your goals.

APPS AND ONLINE TOOLS

Keto Macro Calculators: tasteaholics.com/keto-calculator The simplest and most straightforward.

keto-calculator.ankerl.com The most detailed and complex.

ketogains.com/ketogains-calculator A simple calculator with no charts and only numbers.

MyFitnessPal (app) A diet and exercise journal which provides meal tracking, calorie and macronutrient tracking, automatic calculation of meal nutrition, exercise tracking and caloric spend, and much more.

REFERENCES

Allen, B. G., S. K. Bhatia, J. M. Buatti, K. E. Brandt, et al. "Ketogenic Diets Enhance Oxidative Stress and Radio-Chemo-Therapy Responses in Lung Cancer Xenografts." *Clinical Cancer Research* 19, no. 14 (July 2013): 3905–13. doi:10.1158/1078-0432.

Allen, Bryan G., Sudershan K. Bhatia, Carryn M. Anderson, Julie M. Eichenberger-Gilmore, et al. "Ketogenic Diets as an Adjuvant Cancer Therapy: History and Potential Mechanism." *Redox Biology* vol. 2 (2014): 963–70. doi:10.1016/j.redox.2014.08.002.

Aude, Y., A. S., Agatston, F. Lopez-Jimenez, et al. "The National Cholesterol Education Program Diet vs a Diet Lower in Carbohydrates and Higher in Protein and Monounsaturated Fat: A Randomized Trial." *JAMA Internal Medicine* 164, no. 19 (2004): 2141–46. doi: 10.1001/archinte.164.19.2141.

Brehm, Bonnie J., Randy J. Seeley, Stephen R. Daniels, and David A. D'Alessio. "A Randomized Trial Comparing a Very Low Carbohydrate Diet and a Calorie-Restricted Low Fat Diet on Body Weight and Cardiovascular Risk Factors in Healthy Women." *The Journal of Clinical Endocrinology & Metabolism* 88, no. 4 (January 2009). doi: 10.1210/jc.2002-021480.

Brinkworth, Grant D., Manny Noakes, Jonathan D. Buckley, Jennifer B. Keogh, and Peter M. Clifton. "Long-Term Effects of a Very-Low-Carbohydrate Weight Loss Diet Compared with an Isocaloric Low-Fat Diet after 12 Mo." *The American Journal of Clinical Nutrition* 90, no. 1 (July 2009): 23–32. doi:10.3945/ajcn.2008.27326.

Chowdhury, R., S. Warnakula, S. Kunutsor, F. Crowe, H. A. Ward, et al. "Association of Dietary, Circulating, and Supplement Fatty Acids with Coronary Risk: A Systematic Review and Meta-Analysis." *Annals of Internal Medicine* 160 (2014): 398–406. doi:10.7326/M13-1788.

Daly, M. E., R. Paisey, R. Paisey, B. A. Millward, et al. "Short-Term Effects of Severe Dietary Carbohydrate-Restriction Advice in Type 2 Diabetes—a Randomized Controlled Trial." *Diabetic Medicine* 23, no. 1 (January 2006): 15–20. doi:10.1111/j.1464-5491.2005.01760.x.

Davis, C., and E. Saltos. "Dietary Recommendations and How They Have Changed Over Time," Agriculture Information Bulletin No. (AIB-750) 494 pp, *U.S. Department of Agriculture*, May 1999: 36-44.

De Lau, L. M., M. Bornebroek, J. C. Witteman, A. Hofman, et al. "Dietary Fatty Acids and the Risk of Parkinson Disease: The Rotterdam Study." *Neurology* 64, no. 12 (June 2005): 2040–45. doi:10.1212/01.WNL.0000166038.67153.9F.

Freeman, J. M., E. P. Vining, D. J. Pillas, P. L. Pyzik, et al. "The Efficacy of the Ketogenic Diet-1998: A Prospective Evaluation of Intervention in 150 Children." *Pediatrics* 102, no. 6 (December 1998): 1358–63. www.ncbi.nlm.nih.gov/pubmed/9832569/.

Fryar, C. D., M. D. Carroll, and C. L. Ogden. "Prevalence of Overweight, Obesity, and Extreme Obesity Among Adults: United States, 1960-1962 Through 2011 -2012." Centers for Disease Control and Prevention, September 2014. www.cdc.gov/nchs/data/hestat/obesity_adult_11_12/obesity_adult_11_12.htm#table2.

Hemingway, C., J. M. Freeman, D. J. Pillas, and P. L. Pyzik. "The Ketogenic Diet: A 3- to 6-Year Follow-Up of 150 Children Enrolled Prospectively. *Pediatrics* 108, no. 4 (October 2001): 898–905. www.ncbi.nlm.nih.gov/pubmed/11581442/.

Henderson, S. T. "High Carbohydrate Diets and Alzheimer's Disease." *Medical Hypotheses* 62, no. 5 (2014): 689–700. doi:10.1016/j.mehy.2003.11.028.

Neal, E. G., H. Chaffe, R. H. Schwartz, M. S. Lawson, et al. "The Ketogenic Diet for the Treatment of Childhood Epilepsy: A Randomised Controlled Trial." *Lancet Neurology* 7, no. 6 (June 2008): 500–06. doi:10.1016/S1474-4422(08)70092-9.

Otto, C., U. Kaemmerer, B. Illert, B. Muehling, et al. "Growth of Human Gastric Cancer Cells in Nude Mice Is Delayed by a Ketogenic Diet Supplemented with Omega-3 Fatty Acids and Medium-Chain Triglycerides." *BMC Cancer* 8 (April 2008): 122. doi:10.1186/1471-2407-8-122.

Paoli, Antonio, Antonino Bianco, Ernesto Damiani, and Gerardo Basco. "Ketogenic Diet in Neuromuscular and Neurodegenerative Diseases." *Biomed Research International* 474296 (2014). doi:10.1155/2014/474296.

Samaha, Frederick F., Nayyar Iqbal, Prakash Seshadri, Kathryn L. Chicano, et al. "A Low-Carbohydrate as Compared with a Low-Fat Diet in Severe Obesity." *The New England Journal of Medicine* 348 (May 2003): 2075–81. doi:10.1056/NEJMoa022637.

Siri-Tarino, P. W., Q. Sun, F. B. Hu, and R. M. Krauss. "Meta-Analysis of Prospective Cohort Studies Evaluating the Association of Saturated Fat with Cardiovascular Disease." *American Journal of Clinical Nutrition* 91, no. 3 (March 2010): 535–46. doi:10.3945/ajcn.2009.27725.

Sondike, Stephen B., Nancy Copperman, and Marc S. Jacobson. "Effects of a Low-Carbohydrate Diet on Weight Loss and Cardiovascular Risk Factor in Overweight Adolescents." *The Journal of Pediatrics* 142, no. 3 (March 2003): 253–58. doi: 10.1067/mpd.2003.4.

"Statistics About Diabetes." American Diabetes Association. www.diabetes.org/diabetes-basics/statistics/.

Tetzloff, W., F. Dauchy, S. Medimagh, D. Carr, A. Bärr. "Tolerance to Subchronic, High-Dose Ingestion of Erythritol in Human Volunteers." *Regulatory Toxicology and Pharmacology* 24, no, 2 (October 1996): S286–95. doi:10.1006/rtph.1996.0110.

Vanitallie, T. B., C. Nonas, A. Di Rocco, K. Boyar, S. B. Heymsfield. "Treatment of Parkinson Disease with Diet-Induced Hyperketonemia: A Feasibility Study." *Neurology* 64, no. 4 (February 2005): 728–30. doi:10.1212/01.WNL.0000152046.11390.45.

Volek, J. S., S. D. Phinney, C. E. Forsythe, et al. "Carbohydrate Restriction Has a More Favorable Impact on the Metabolic Syndrome than a Low Fat Diet." *Lipids* 44, no. 4 (2009): 297. doi:10.1007/s11745-008-3274-2.

Volek, J. S., M. J. Sharman, A. L. Gómez, D. A. Judelson, et al. "Comparison of Energy-Restricted Very Low-Carbohydrate and Low-Fat Diets on Weight Loss and Body Composition in Overweight Men and Women." *Nutrition & Metabolism* 1 (2004): 13. doi: 10.1186/1743-7075-1-13.

Westman, Eric C., William S. Yancy, John C. Mavropoulos, Megan Marquart, and Jennifer R. McDuffie. "The Effect of a Low-Carbohydrate, Ketogenic Diet versus a Low-Glycemic Index Diet on Glycemic Control in Type 2 Diabetes Mellitus." *Nutrition & Metabolism* 5 (2008): 36. doi:10.1186/1743-7075-5-36.

Zuccoli, G., N. Marcello, A. Pisanello, F. Servadei, et al. "Metabolic Management of Glioblastoma Multiforme Using Standard Therapy Together with a Restricted Ketogenic Diet: Case Report." *Nutrition & Metabolism* 7 (2010): 33. doi:10.1186/1743-7075-7-33.

RECIPE INDEX

INDEX

CPSIA information can be obtained
at www.ICGtesting.com
Printed in the USA
BVHW051350090819
555473BV00001BA/1/P